EMBRYOLOGY
COLOURING BOOK

George Matsumura

Associate Professor of Anatomy,
Hokkaido University School of Medicine,
Sapporo, Japan

Marjorie A. England

Senior Lecturer in Anatomy,
Medical Sciences,
University of Leicester,
Leicester, UK

and lately

Honorary Senior Research Fellow,
Royal College of Surgeons of England

Mosby

MOSBY
An imprint of Harcourt Publishers Limited

Copyright © 1992 Mosby-Year Book Limited
Copyright © 1999 Harcourt Publishers Limited
Printed by Grafos, Arte Sobre Papel, Barcelona, Spain
ISBN 0 7234 1883 7
First published 1992
Reprinted 1994
Reprinted 1999

In Honour of

Professor H. Nishimura, Kyoto
and the Late

Professor A. d'A. Bellairs, London

Contents

Preface

Embryology can be a difficult subject for many students and there are two major obstacles to success. Firstly, it may require long hours of study to acquire the ability to visualise a developing embryo in three dimensions. Secondly, there is a need to master a new and large vocabulary to describe these developmental processes. Students, however, often lack the time to deal with a single subject in such depth.

Both of these problems can be solved by the use of a shortened text and labelled diagrams to be coloured by the student.

This book has been designed to present a short and concise text which is manageable but contains the required information.

The illustrations are intended to aid an understanding of normal embryological development. Space has only permitted certain abnormalities to be illustrated; others are described in the text.

Diagrams to be coloured by the student provide opportunities for actively participating in the learning process. A clear understanding of the development of a structure will result from colouring a sequence through its three dimensional development. As the diagrams are labelled, the reader will learn their names while colouring and can refer to the text for further information. Everyone enjoys colouring, whatever their age, and this technique provides an enjoyable method of learning a difficult subject, as well as stimulating curiosity and further understanding.

It is suggested that coloured pencils be used rather than felt tip pens. The colours and their abbreviations are as follows:

Red	R
dark Red	dR
light Blue	lB
dark Blue	dB
Yellow	Y
light Green	lG
dark Green	dG
Brown	B
Purple	P
Orange	O
Pink	Pk

Acknowledgements

The authors are very grateful to Professor Ruth Bellairs, University College London, for reading and commenting upon our book. Her excellent suggestions have improved our work and we are deeply grateful for all her labours. Our meetings with her were both educational and enjoyable and will be remembered with pleasure.

Professor M. Marin-Padilla, Dartmouth College, USA, kindly advised us on **40**. Histology of the Cerebral Cortex, and we are grateful for his help. Dr Brian Wilkins, University of Leicester, suggested alterations to **121**. Congenital Malformations, and we are pleased to thank him for his corrections. We also appreciate the assistance given by Dr Jennifer Wakely, University of Leicester, who kindly read the manuscript and commented upon it.

We are also pleased to thank Mr I. Indans, University of Leicester, who commented upon those sections concerned with implantation and placentation. Mr G. L. C. McTurk and Dr C. G. Page, University of Leicester, kindly advised us on computer usage. Miss D. Meecham, University of Leicester, assisted us with some alterations to the drawings. Dr J. M. England, Consultant Haematologist, Watford General Hospital, also read and corrected the original manuscript and we are grateful for all his work and efforts.

Mrs L. Bradshaw cheerfully typed and produced the manuscript to a very high standard. We are indebted to her for all her work.

The authors are very pleased to thank Lara Last, Caroline Turner and Rosemary Watts, Wolfe Publishing, for their patience and assistance during the publication of this book.

INTRODUCTION TO EMBRYOLOGY

1. Terminology

Directions

The top of the embryo or fetus' head is referred to as cranial, superior, or cephalic, and the rump end is caudal or inferior.

The embryo's back is dorsal and the belly-side is ventral. The midline is referred to as medial, while toward the nose is rostral.

Plane of Section

Embryos and fetuses are usually sectioned in one of three planes: longitudinally (median or sagittal); coronal (frontal); and transverse (horizontal). Very early embryos are usually in a flexed position and a transverse section may include both the head and tail in the same plane.

INTRODUCTION TO EMBRYOLOGY

1. TERMINOLOGY

DIRECTIONS (R)

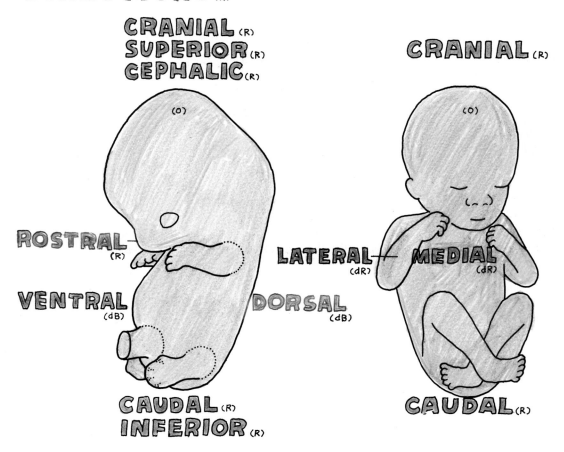

CRANIAL (R)
SUPERIOR (R)
CEPHALIC (R)

(O)

ROSTRAL (R)

VENTRAL (dB)

DORSAL (dB)

CAUDAL (R)
INFERIOR (R)

CRANIAL (R)

(O)

LATERAL (dR) — MEDIAL (dR)

CAUDAL (R)

PLANE OF SECTION (PR)

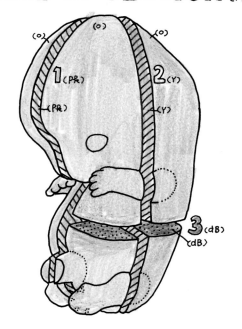

(O)   (O)   (O)

1 (PR)   2 (Y)

(PR)   (Y)

3 (dB)
(dB)

1 LONGITUDINAL (PR)
   (MEDIAN / SAGITTAL)
2 CORONAL (Y)
   (FRONTAL)
3 TRANSVERSE (dB)
   (HORIZONTAL)

Embryonic Staging

Estimated ages of embryos and fetuses are based on a series of developing features and organs summarised in *Developmental Stages in Human Embryos*, e.g. Carnegie Stage 10, which is at Day 22 and when the heart begins to beat. Older methods of ageing include the crown–rump (CR) measurement, which is made in a straight line from the crown of the embryo's head to its rump. In older fetuses, the crown–heel (CH) measurement was made by taking the CR measurement and adding the length of the leg down to the heel. These estimates of age, based solely on linear measurement, may be unreliable because of handling, fixation, etc., when specimens are preserved.

EMBRYONIC STAGING (R)

CARNEGIE STAGE (R)

11　12　15　17　19　20　23

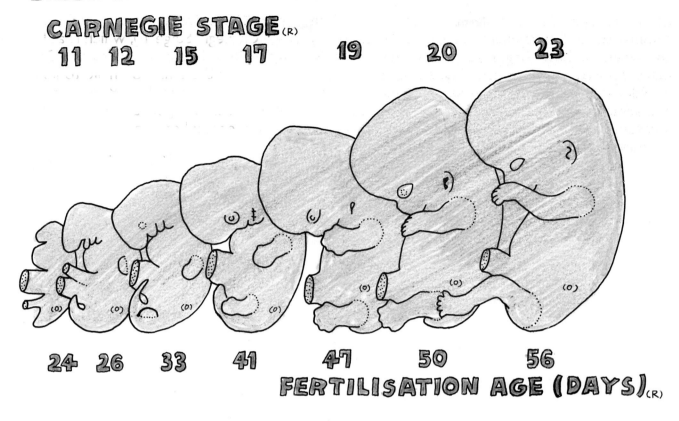

24　26　33　41　47　50　56

FERTILISATION AGE (DAYS) (R)

MEASUREMENT (R)

CR: CROWN-RUMP (R)　　CH: CROWN-HEEL (R)

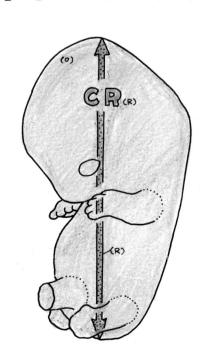

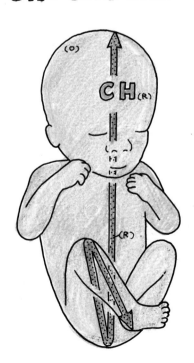

15

2. General Development: Pre- and Embryonic Period

The period of gestation is from fertilisation time 0 (Stage 1, true age) to term at Week 38 (Day 266). Medical practitioners divide this period into trimesters, each of 3 months duration. Measurements made using ultrasound allow a fertilisation date to be assigned with an accuracy of 1–2 days. Older methods based on menstrual age or lunar months are not as accurate.

This gestational period can also be divided into the pre-embryonic period (Carnegie Stages 1–8); the embryonic period, which ends at Week 8 (Stages 9–23); and the fetal period, which extends from the end of the second month to Week 38.

The pre-embryonic period includes fertilisation, implantation, and the formation of the trilaminar embryo. All of the basic organs and systems are laid down during the embryonic period. This period ends at the end of Week 8 (Stage 23).

2. GENERAL DEVELOPMENT:
PRE- AND EMBRYONIC PERIOD

DAYS (G)

FERTILISATION AGE (WEEKS)

DAYS			
1 (G)	STAGE 1 (dB)	FERTILISATION (dR)	
		UNICELLULAR (dR)	
4	STAGE 3 (dB)	FREE BLASTOCYST (R)	
7	STAGE 5 (dB)	IMPLANTATION	
13	STAGE 6 (dB)	CHORIONIC VILLI (PR)	
		PRIMITIVE STREAK (PR)	
16	STAGE 7 (dB)	NOTOCHORDAL PROCESS	
22	STAGE 10 (dB)	SOMITES (dR)	
		HEART BEATS (dR)	
24	STAGE 11 (dB)	OPTIC VESICLE	
28	STAGE 13 (dB)	FOUR LIMB BUDS (R)	
32	STAGE 14 (dB)	LENS PIT (lB)	
33	STAGE 15 (dB)	HAND PLATE	
37	STAGE 16 (dB)		
		FOOT PLATE	
41	STAGE 17 (dB)		
		FINGER RAYS (PR)	
44	STAGE 18 (dB)	TOE RAYS (PR)	
		NIPPLES (PR)	
50	STAGE 20 (dB)		
		ELBOWS BEND (Y)	
56	STAGE 23 (dB)		
		HEAD ROUNDED (dR)	
		LIMBS LONGER (dR)	

STAGE 1 (dR)

STAGE 3 (R)

STAGE 6 (PR)

STAGE 10 (O) (dR)

STAGE 13 (O) (R)

STAGE 14 (O) (lB)

STAGE 17 (O) (PR)

STAGE 18 (O) (PR)

STAGE 20 (O) (Y)

STAGE 23 (O)

17

3. General Development: Fetal Period

The fetus has a human appearance and the name in Greek means 'young one'. During the fetal period (Weeks 9–38), the fetus develops further and grows very rapidly with a dramatic increase in weight in the final months.

Fetal movements are first detected at Week 7, although the mother will not be aware of them until Weeks 16–20. These movements are referred to as 'quickening'. In the fourth month, a white protective coating, the *vernix caseosa* covers the skin. By Week 20, a fine hair called lanugo, covers most of the body. This is shed in Weeks 35–38 or shortly after birth.

Fetuses born from Week 25 onwards may survive with appropriate medical care (see **68**. Histological Stages of Lung Development).

3. GENERAL DEVELOPMENT : FETAL PERIOD

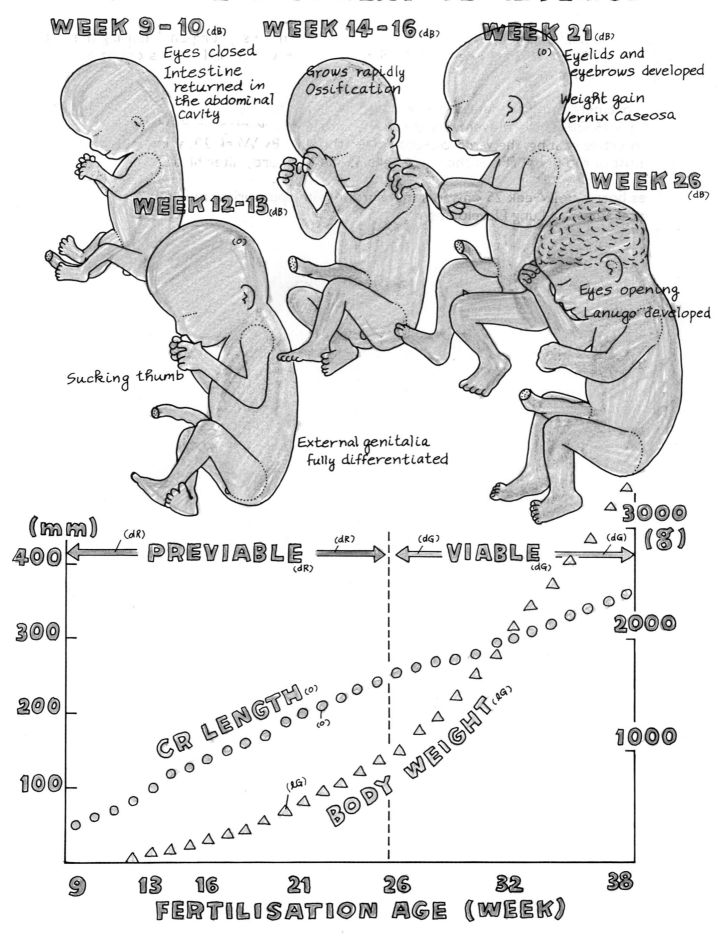

WEEK 9-10 (dB)

Eyes closed
Intestine returned in the abdominal cavity

WEEK 14-16 (dB)

Grows rapidly
Ossification

WEEK 21 (dB)

(o) Eyelids and eyebrows developed

Weight gain
Vernix Caseosa

WEEK 12-13 (dB)

(o)

Sucking thumb

External genitalia fully differentiated

WEEK 26 (dB)

Eyes opening
Lanugo developed

(mm)

400

PREVIABLE (dR) → ← VIABLE → (dG)

(g)

3000

CR LENGTH (o)

(o)

BODY WEIGHT (ᴸG)

(ᴸG)

300   2000

200   1000

100

9   13   16   21   26   32   38

FERTILISATION AGE (WEEK)

EARLY DEVELOPMENT

4. Fertilisation

The fusion of the male and female germ cells (sperm and secondary oocyte) results in the formation of a new individual. This process is referred to as fertilisation or conception. The fusion of the male and female pronuclei (haploid nuclei) results in the diploid number (46 chromosomes) being restored, as well as the chromosomal sex of the individual being established.

During sexual intercourse, between 300–500 million sperm are normally ejaculated by the male into the female vagina. They then traverse the cervix, uterus, and uterine tubes where fertilisation occurs in the expanded portion of the tube called the ampulla. The secondary oocyte is fertilised 12–24 hours after ovulation although sperm are capable of fertilisation for 2–3 days.

As the sperm approach the secondary oocyte, the acrosomal reaction of the sperm head is initiated. Hyaluronidase is released and causes the corona radiata cells to separate from the secondary oocyte, and the release of neuraminidase and acrosin facilitates the entry of a sperm through the zona pellucida. As soon as a sperm penetrates the thick zona pellucida and contacts the plasma membrane of the secondary oocyte, the zonal reaction prevents any further sperm from penetrating the secondary oocyte. The secondary oocyte then completes its second meiotic division resulting in the production of the second polar body. The secondary oocyte is now referred to as a mature ovum and its nucleus as the female pronucleus.

Following the sperm's entry into the ovum, it loses its tail, and its head enlarges to form the male pronucleus which then fuses with the female pronucleus. The chromosomes of the two pronuclei intermingle to form the new unique individual. This cell is now referred to as a zygote.

The zygote undergoes rapid mitotic cell divisions (cleavage) during a period of approximately two more days during which it travels from the uterine tube to the uterus. The newly formed cells are known as blastomeres. With each cell division the individual cells become smaller in size. Eventually a ball of 16 cells is formed, called the morula.

As the morula enters the uterus, it draws in uterine fluid and fluid-filled spaces appear. The spaces fuse to form a large central fluid-filled blastocyst cavity and the morula is now known as a blastocyst. The flattened cells around its perimeter form the walls of the ball. These cells are known as the trophoblast and will eventually become the embryonic contribution to the placenta. At one end of the hollow ball of cells is a group of cells known as the inner cell mass which will eventually form the embryo.

By Day 6 the blastocyst will begin to implant in the uterus.

A low sperm count (below 20 million/ml with only 40% of sperm being motile) is one cause of male infertility. If the uterine tubes are blocked, fertilisation is unable to occur normally.

EARLY DEVELOPMENT

4. FERTILISATION

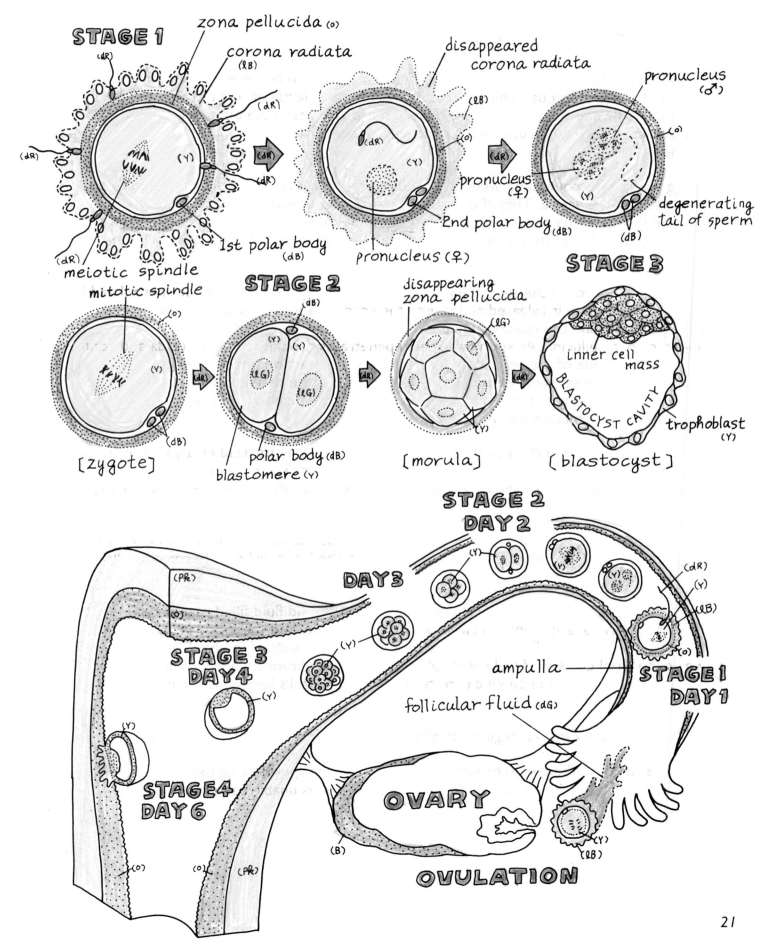

STAGE 1
zona pellucida (O)
corona radiata (lB)
(dR)
(dR)
(dR)
(dR)
(Y)
1st polar body (dB)
meiotic spindle
mitotic spindle

disappeared corona radiata
(dR)
(Y)
(lB)
2nd polar body (dB)
pronucleus (♀)

pronucleus (♂)
(O)
pronucleus (♀)
(Y)
(dB)
degenerating tail of sperm

STAGE 3

(O)
(Y)
(dB)
[zygote]

STAGE 2
(dB)
(Y)
(Y)
(lG)
(lG)
polar body (dB)
blastomere (Y)

disappearing zona pellucida
(lG)
(Y)
[morula]

inner cell mass
BLASTOCYST CAVITY
trophoblast (Y)
[blastocyst]

STAGE 2 DAY 2

DAY 3
(Y)
(Y)
(Y)
(dR)
(Y)
(lB)
(O)

(Prk)
(O)
STAGE 3 DAY 4
(Y)
(Y)
ampulla
follicular fluid (dG)
STAGE 1 DAY 1

(Y)
STAGE 4 DAY 6
OVARY
(B)
(Y)
(lB)
(O)
(O)
(Prk)
OVULATION

21

5. Early Stage of Implantation

The blastocyst normally embeds in the dorsal wall of the body of the uterus. By Day 5, the zona pellucida disappears, and the trophoblast layer of the blastocyst contacts and becomes attached to the maternal endometrium by Day 6. The attached trophoblast differentiates to form two layers: an outer syncytiotrophoblast in direct contact with the maternal tissue, and an inner cytotrophoblast. The syncytiotrophoblast is a syncytium where the cytotrophoblast cells have fused to form a multinucleated layer.

By Day 7, the ventral-most cells of the inner cell mass have differentiated to form the hypoblast layer or embryonic endoderm layer. This is the first germ layer to form in the embryo and is the beginning of embryogenesis. The formation of the three embryonic germ layers (ectoderm, mesoderm, and endoderm) is called gastrulation. These three layers will ultimately give rise to all the tissues in the body. The remaining inner cell mass will form the second germ layer of epiblast or embryonic ectoderm in Week 2. The third layer, the mesoblast or embryonic mesoderm, forms in Week 3.

Implantation occurring outside the uterus, i.e. in the uterine tubes or abdominal cavity, is referred to as an ectopic pregnancy. If such a pregnancy proceeds, it will result in serious complications.

5. EARLY STAGE OF IMPLANTATION
STAGE 4   ATTACHING BLASTOCYST
(DAY 6)

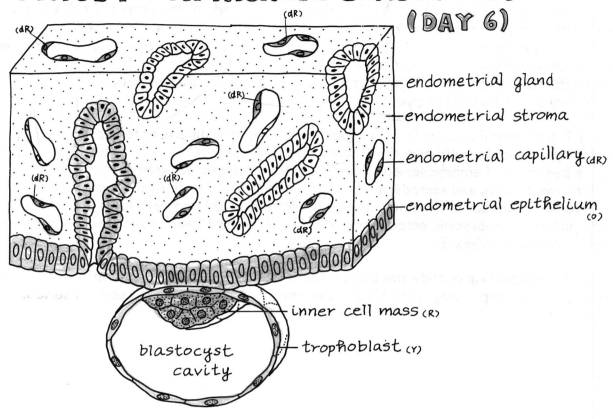

endometrial gland

endometrial stroma

endometrial capillary (dR)

endometrial epithelium (o)

inner cell mass (R)

trophoblast (Y)

blastocyst cavity

STAGE 4   BEGINNING OF IMPLANTATION
(DAY 7)

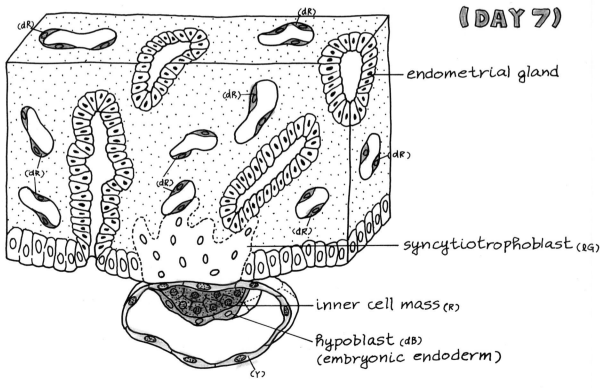

endometrial gland

syncytiotrophoblast (lG)

inner cell mass (R)

hypoblast (dB)
(embryonic endoderm)

6. Late Stage of Implantation

During Stage 5 (Week 2) the blastocyst implants and gradually becomes completely embedded in the maternal endometrium by Day 10. A fibrin clot (closing plug) marks the site of implantation for 1 or 2 days before the maternal epithelium regenerates.

   As more and more of the blastocyst's trophoblast contacts the maternal tissue, it differentiates to form syncytiotrophoblast and cytotrophoblast layers. As the blastocyst invades the maternal epithelium, the syncytiotrophoblast contacts and erodes the uterine glands and maternal blood vessels. Lacunae (lakes) form of maternal blood, uterine secretion, and cell debris; these provide the blastocyst with nourishment. A primitive uteroplacental circulation is established as the lacunae link-up to form lacunar networks through which the maternal blood flows. This circulation provides the early embryo with nutrients and oxygen, and removes waste products and carbon dioxide. (By the end of Week 2, outgrowths from the trophoblast have formed primary chorionic villi which will contribute to the formation of the placenta (see **15**. Amniotic Sac and Chorion).)

6. LATE STAGE OF IMPLANTATION

STAGE 5 (sagittal section)

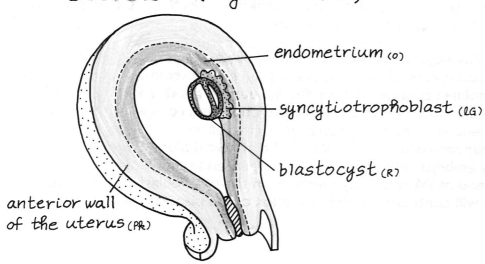

endometrium (O)

syncytiotrophoblast (LG)

blastocyst (R)

anterior wall
of the uterus (PK)

STAGE 5 (DAY 8)

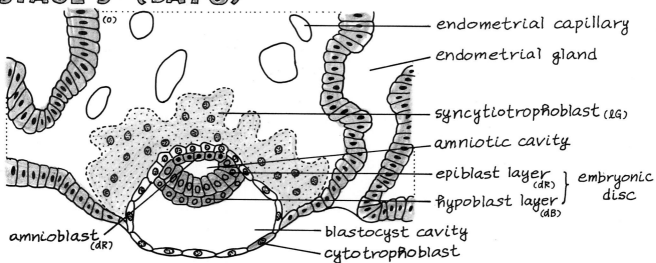

(O)

endometrial capillary

endometrial gland

syncytiotrophoblast (LG)

amniotic cavity

epiblast layer (dR) } embryonic
disc

hypoblast layer (dB)

blastocyst cavity

cytotrophoblast

amnioblast (dR)

STAGE 5 (DAY 8-9)

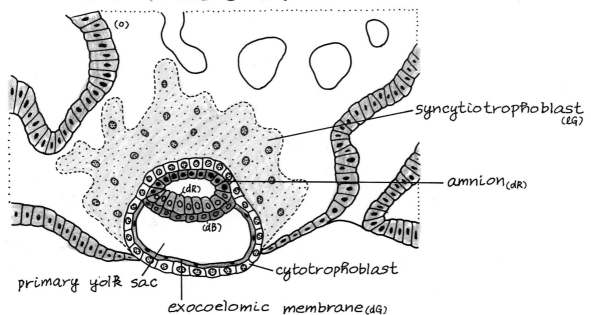

(O)

syncytiotrophoblast (LG)

amnion (dR)

(dR)

(dB)

primary yolk sac

cytotrophoblast

exocoelomic membrane (dG)

Embryonic Disc

During implantation, the inner cell mass further differentiates to form the amnion and amniotic cavity, and the epiblast layer.

Early in Week 2, a cleft appears between the inner cell mass and the cytotrophoblastic layer; this marks the site of the future amniotic cavity. At the same time, the inner cell mass differentiates to form an epiblast layer which faces the future amniotic cavity dorsally and contacts the hypoblast layer ventrally. The early embryo is now a bilaminar embryonic disc with two germ cell layers: epiblast and hypoblast.

STAGE 5 (DAY 9)

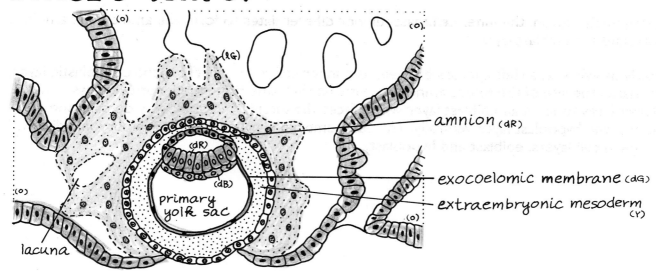

amnion (dR)

exocoelomic membrane (dG)

extraembryonic mesoderm (Y)

primary yolk sac

lacuna

STAGE 5 (DAY 10)

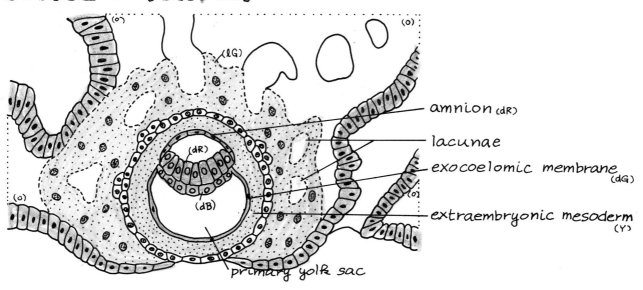

amnion (dR)

lacunae

exocoelomic membrane (dG)

extraembryonic mesoderm (Y)

primary yolk sac

Primary Yolk Sac

As the amnion forms, cells from the cytotrophoblast differentiate to form an exocoelomic membrane which becomes the wall of the primary yolk sac. The exocoelomic membrane is continuous with the embryonic hypoblast layer (see **14**. Yolk Sac and Allantois).

STAGE 5 (DAY 12)

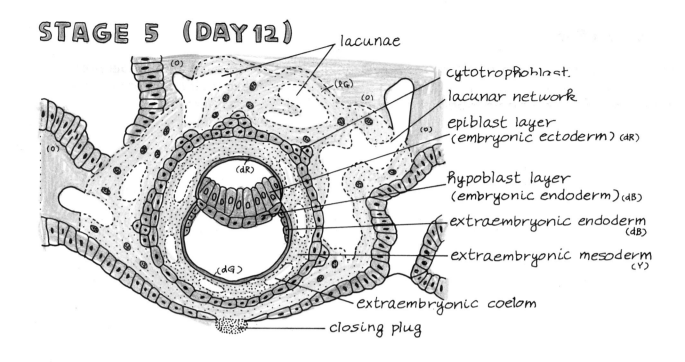

lacunae

cytotrophoblast

lacunar network

epiblast layer
(embryonic ectoderm) (dR)

hypoblast layer
(embryonic endoderm) (dB)

extraembryonic endoderm
(dB)

extraembryonic mesoderm
(Y)

extraembryonic coelom

closing plug

STAGE 6 (DAY 13)

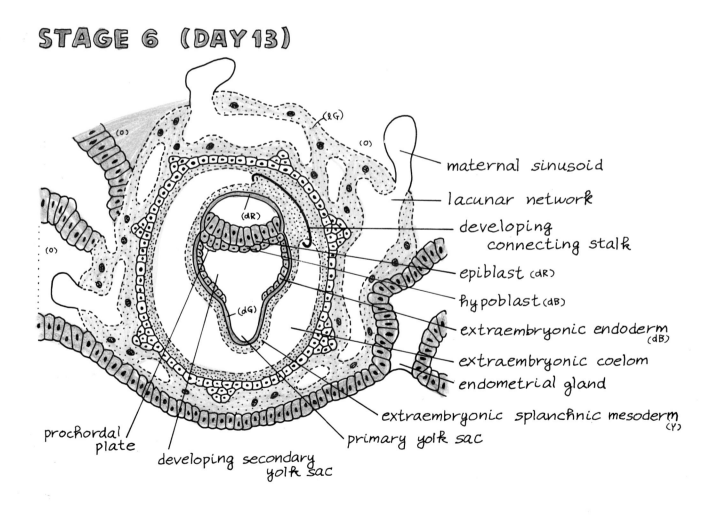

maternal sinusoid

lacunar network

developing
connecting stalk

epiblast (dR)

hypoblast (dB)

extraembryonic endoderm
(dB)

extraembryonic coelom

endometrial gland

extraembryonic splanchnic mesoderm
(Y)

primary yolk sac

developing secondary
yolk sac

prochordal
plate

7. Primitive Streak

With the formation of the primitive streak, the third germ layer, the intraembryonic mesoderm, develops. The formation of the three germ layers (epiblast, mesoblast, and hypoblast) is known as gastrulation and is completed in Weeks 3–4. The bilaminar embryonic disc is converted into a trilaminar embryonic disc in Week 3.

In Week 3, the epiblast thickens in the future caudal region of the embryo. This midline thickening forms a rod-like shape as it increases in length and elongates to reach the middle of the embryonic disc. This is the primitive streak and demarcates for the first time, the embryonic cephalic, caudal, right and left sides of the future embryo.

When the streak reaches its greatest length, a mound of cells called the primitive knot develops together with a primitive pit at the cephalic end of the streak. A midline primitive groove is present in the primitive streak.

With the expansion of the embryonic disc, epiblast cells migrate as a layer towards the primitive streak. Upon reaching the primitive groove, the epiblast cells migrate ventrally through the groove to enter the space between the epiblast and the hypoblast. Entering this space, they form the third germ layer, the mesoblast (or mesenchyme). The majority of these cells migrate laterally as the mesoderm layer. They also migrate cephalically and caudally except into the region of the prochordal plate and cloacal membrane (future anal membrane). Some of the mesoblast cells enter the hypoblast layer directly to displace these cells laterally. These newly-added mesoblast cells form the embryonic endoderm. The epiblast cells which did not invaginate through the primitive streak remain as the embryonic ectoderm layer.

7. PRIMITIVE STREAK
STAGE 6 (sagittal section)

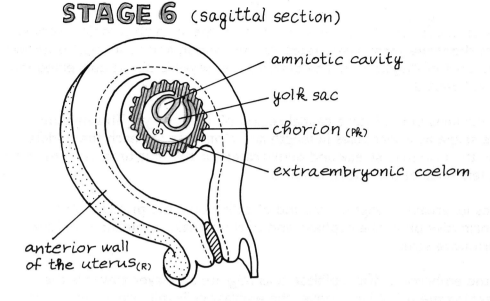

amniotic cavity

yolk sac

chorion (Pk)

extraembryonic coelom

anterior wall of the uterus(R)

STAGE 6

STAGE 6

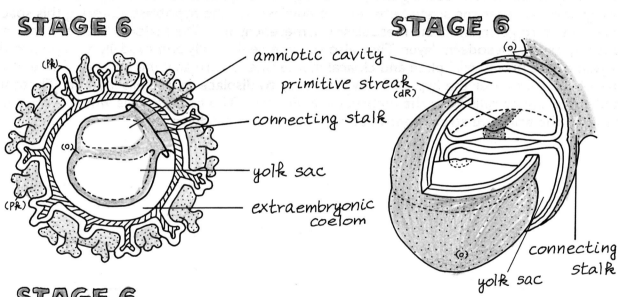

amniotic cavity

primitive streak (dR)

connecting stalk

yolk sac

extraembryonic coelom

connecting stalk

yolk sac

STAGE 6

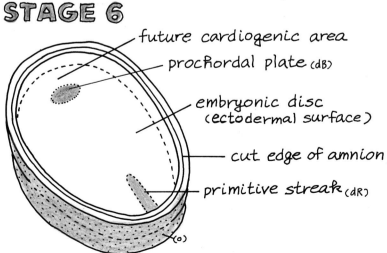

future cardiogenic area

prochordal plate (dB)

embryonic disc (ectodermal surface)

cut edge of amnion

primitive streak (dR)

Cephalic to the primitive knot, the prochordal plate demarcates the area of the future oropharyngeal membrane and mouth region. No mesoblast cells are present in this region. A similar area caudally demarcates the future cloacal membrane. Cephalic to the prochordal plate are the cardiogenic area and the septum transversum. The cardiogenic area is composed of mesenchyme cells which will form the primitive heart. The septum transversum is also a region of mesenchyme cells which will form the ventral mesentery of the liver, contribute to the liver and to the diaphragm later in development.

When the primitive streak has reached its definitive length, the epiblast cells invaginating through the primitive knot and pit form a midline collection of mesoderm cells called the notochordal process. It is the notochordal process and its associated mesoderm which causes or 'induces' the overlying ectoderm to form the neural plate.

STAGE 6-7

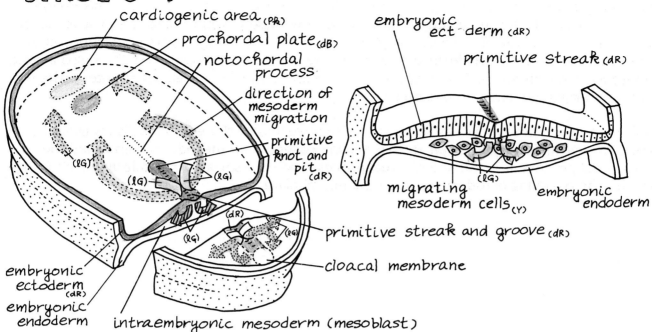

cardiogenic area (PR)

prochordal plate (dB)

notochordal process

direction of mesoderm migration

primitive knot and pit (dR)

(lG)

(lG)

(lG)

(lG)

(dR)

(lG)

embryonic ectoderm (dR)

embryonic endoderm

intraembryonic mesoderm (mesoblast)

embryonic ectoderm (dR)

primitive streak (dR)

migrating mesoderm cells (Y)

(lG)

embryonic endoderm

primitive streak and groove (dR)

cloacal membrane

8. Notochord

The notochord develops in Weeks 3–4. The primitive pit extends into the midline notochordal process and forms a central notochordal canal. The cells of the notochordal process condense around this lumen to form a tube. The notochordal process lengthens cephalically as the embryonic disc lengthens. It then extends from the primitive knot and reaches, but does not enter, the prochordal plate region; here the ectoderm and endoderm layers are in apposition.

As the notochordal process lengthens, the primitive streak regresses laying down more notochordal process in its wake. Eventually in Week 4, the primitive streak reaches the caudal end of the embryonic disc where it ultimately disappears.

As the notochordal process lengthens, its floor fuses with the underlying endoderm layer. The two fused layers degenerate, bringing the notochordal canal and yolk sac into communication. There is now a direct communication between the yolk sac and amniotic cavity via the primitive pit. This communication is called the neurenteric canal.

The remaining dorsal portion of the notochordal process is called the notochordal plate. Cranially, the two lateral edges of the plate bend ventrally and fuse to form a solid, rod-like structure, the notochord. The transformation of the plate proceeds caudally and, when completed, the neurenteric canal normally disappears.

The endoderm layer re-establishes its continuity.

Much later (Weeks 4–7), the vertebral column develops around the notochord. Where the notochord has been incorporated in the vertebral bodies, the notochord degenerates. It persists, however, in the intervertebral discs as the nucleus pulposus of the adult (see **107**. Vertebral Column).

Anomalies of the Primitive Streak

Remnants of the primitive streak can give rise to a sacrococcygeal teratoma or tumour.

8. NOTOCHORD
STAGE 7-8

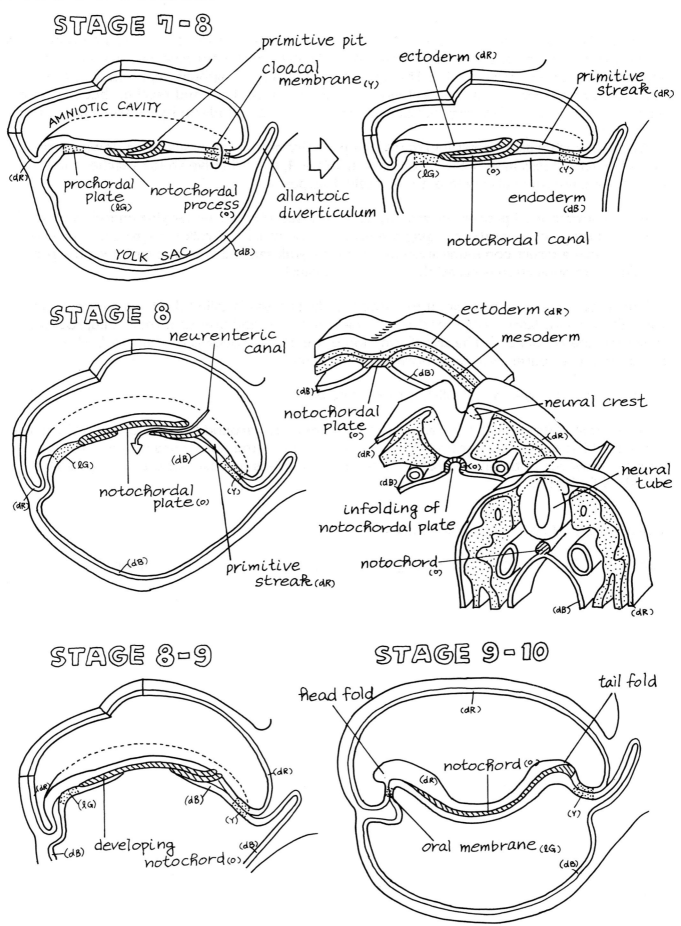

primitive pit

cloacal membrane (Y)

ectoderm (dR)

primitive streak (dR)

AMNIOTIC CAVITY

(dR)

prochordal plate (lG)

notochordal process (o)

allantoic diverticulum

endoderm (dB)

notochordal canal

YOLK SAC (dB)

STAGE 8

neurenteric canal

ectoderm (dR)

mesoderm

(dB)

notochordal plate (o)

neural crest

(dR)

(dR)

(lG)

(dB)

(Y)

notochordal plate (o)

(dR)

(dB)

neural tube

infolding of notochordal plate

notochord (o)

primitive streak (dR)

(dB)

(dR)

STAGE 8-9

(dR)

(dR)

(lG)

(dB)

(Y)

(dB)

developing notochord (o)

(dB)

STAGE 9-10

head fold

tail fold

(dR)

notochord (o)

(dR)

(Y)

oral membrane (lG)

(dB)

9. Neural Plate, Neural Tube, Neural Crest

The neural plate is formed when the ectoderm cephalic to the primitive knot is induced in Week 3 by the underlying notochordal process and its associated mesoderm to form neuroectoderm. This is the first indication of the central nervous system.

A longitudinal groove running cephalocaudally forms in the midline of the neural plate, flanked by two parallel neural folds. The neural folds then elevate and fuse in the median plane opposite somites 2–7 to form the neural tube. Fusion then proceeds both cranially and caudally until only the two ends of the tube remain open, the rostral and caudal neuropores. Eventually they also close; the rostral neuropore on Day 24 and the caudal one approximately 2 days later. The site of the rostral neuropore corresponds to the lamina terminalis of the adult brain. The neural tube cephalic to somite 4 will form the brain and caudal to it will form the spinal cord. As the tube forms, the integrity of the overlying ectoderm layer is re-established.

As the neural folds fuse to form the neural tube, a specialised group of neuroectoderm cells lying between the tube and the overlying ectoderm, the neural crest, separates from them both. The neural crest will migrate throughout the body and have numerous derivatives, e.g. pigment cells, the spinal ganglia, Schwann cells (see 13. Derivatives of the Germ Layers: Ectoderm, Mesoderm and Endoderm).

9. NEURAL PLATE, NEURAL TUBE, NEURAL CREST

STAGE 8   STAGE 8

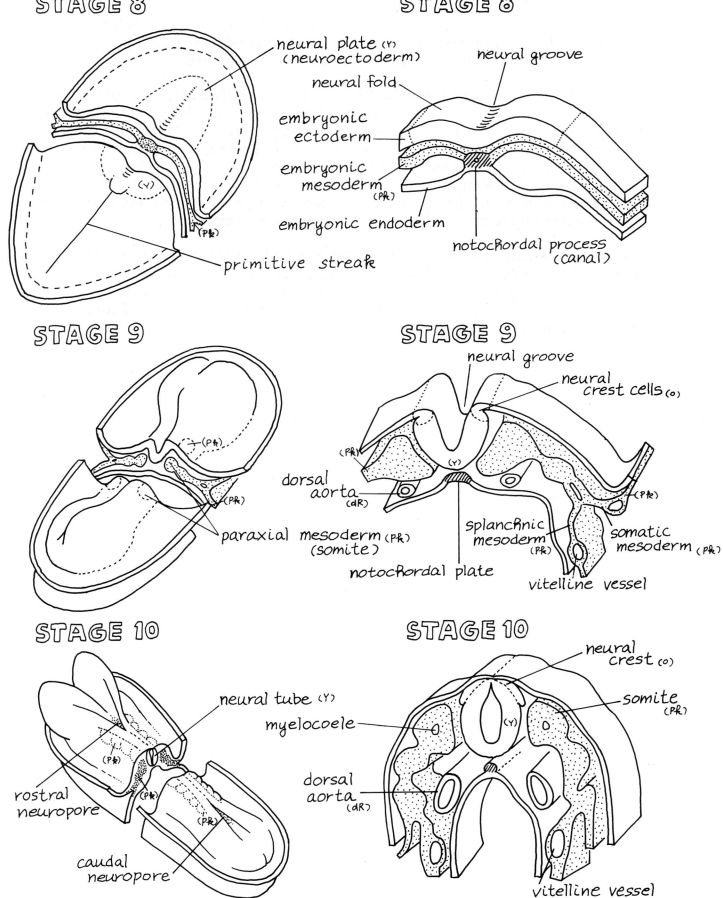

neural plate (Y)
(neuroectoderm)

neural groove

neural fold

embryonic
ectoderm

embryonic
mesoderm
(Pk)

embryonic endoderm

primitive streak

notochordal process
(canal)

STAGE 9   STAGE 9

neural groove

neural
crest cells (o)

(Pk)

(Y)

dorsal
aorta
(dR)

paraxial mesoderm (Pk)
(somite)

splanchnic
mesoderm
(Pk)

somatic
mesoderm (Pk)

notochordal plate

vitelline vessel

STAGE 10   STAGE 10

neural tube (Y)

neural
crest (o)

myelocoele

somite
(Pk)

(Y)

rostral
neuropore

(Pk)

dorsal
aorta
(dR)

caudal
neuropore

vitelline vessel

10. Intraembryonic Coelom

The intraembryonic coelom first forms in the cephalic half of the embryo. Spaces appear in the lateral mesoderm and in the cardiogenic mesoderm which coalesce to form a horseshoe shape. The two ends of the horseshoe are continuous with the extraembryonic coelom.

During the formation of the intraembryonic coelom, the lateral mesoderm is divided into two layers. The first of these is the somatic or somatopleuric mesoderm which is adjacent to the ectoderm layer and is continuous with the extraembryonic mesoderm of the amnion. The second is the splanchnic or splanchnopleuric mesoderm which is adjacent to the endoderm and is continuous with the extraembryonic mesoderm of the yolk sac.

As the head, tail and lateral folds are forming, the intraembryonic coelom is carried into the location where, later, it will form the three main body cavities, i.e. those around the heart (pericardial cavity), the lungs (pleural cavities), and the abdominal and pelvic organs (the peritoneal cavity) (see **61**. Pleuropericardial Membranes, and **62**. Diaphragm (Including Pleuroperitoneal Membranes) Formation).

10. INTRAEMBRYONIC COELOM

STAGE 9

STAGE 9

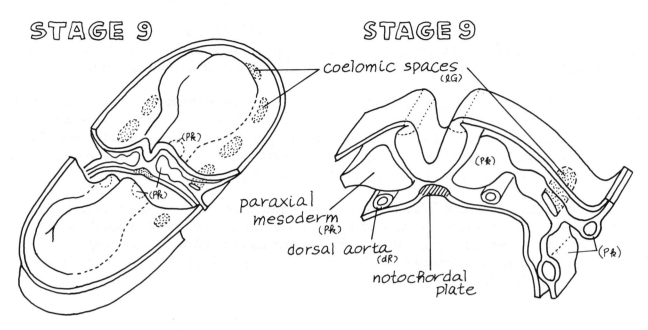

coelomic spaces (ℓG)

paraxial mesoderm (Pk)

dorsal aorta (dR)

notochordal plate

STAGE 10 (4 SOMITES)

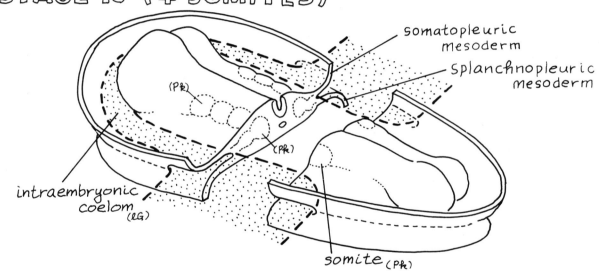

somatopleuric mesoderm

splanchnopleuric mesoderm

intraembryonic coelom (ℓG)

somite (Pk)

STAGE 12

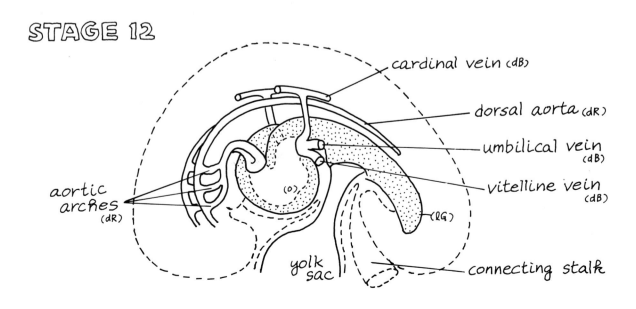

cardinal vein (dB)

dorsal aorta (dR)

umbilical vein (dB)

vitelline vein (dB)

aortic arches (dR)

yolk sac

connecting stalk

11. Somites

Mesoderm immediately adjacent to the embryonic axis forms a longitudinal column on either side. This column is called the paraxial mesoderm. Between Days 20–30, the paraxial mesoderm on either side divides into cubes to form approximately 38 pairs of somites. Laterally, the somites remain continuous with the intermediate mesoderm. The total number formed is between 42–44 somites and their numbers are useful in staging embryos.

Each somite is composed of two major cell populations: the sclerotome and the dermomyotome and these are organised around a central cavity known as the myocoele. The cells from the sclerotome will migrate to surround the notochord and contribute to the vertebral column and ribs. The dermomyotome will give rise to two main derivatives: the dermatome region will form the dermal layer of the skin and the myotome region will form the muscles of the back. The myocoele disappears.

11. SOMITES
STAGE 8 (PRESOMITE STAGE)

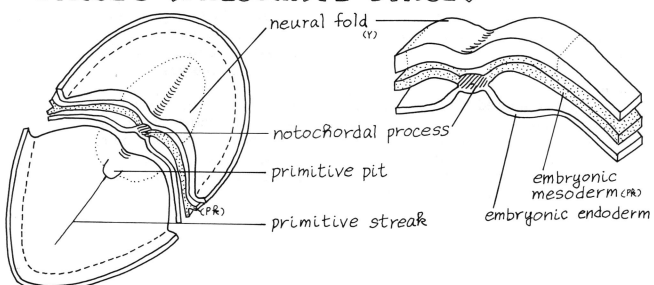

neural fold (Y)

notochordal process

primitive pit

primitive streak

(PR)

embryonic mesoderm (PR)

embryonic endoderm

STAGE 9 (EARLY SOMITE STAGE)

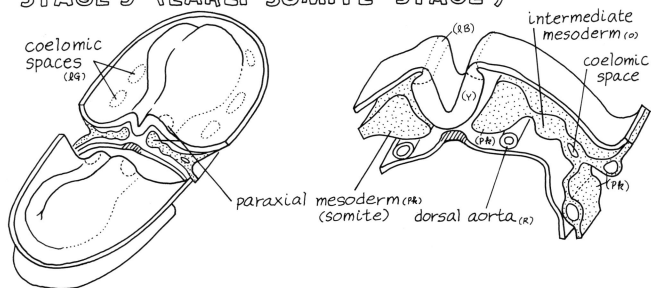

coelomic spaces (lG)

intermediate mesoderm (o)

coelomic space

(lB)

(Y)

(PR)

(PR)

paraxial mesoderm (PR) (somite)

dorsal aorta (R)

STAGE 10

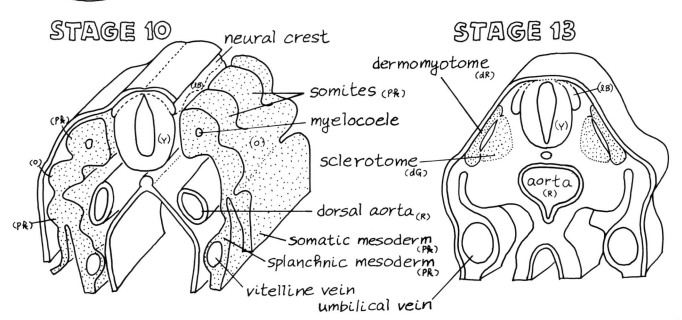

neural crest

somites (PR)

myelocoele

dermomyotome (dR)

sclerotome (dG)

dorsal aorta (R)

somatic mesoderm (PR)

splanchnic mesoderm (PR)

vitelline vein

umbilical vein

STAGE 13

aorta (R)

(lB)

(Y)

12. Head and Tail Folds

In Week 4, the bilaminar, flattened embryonic disc folds ventrally in a continuous sequence. As the head, tail and two lateral folds form ventrally, they incorporate the dorsal part of the yolk sac and constrict it to form the yolk stalk.

That portion of the yolk sac in the head fold forms the embryonic foregut, while that portion in the tail fold forms the embryonic hindgut. The oropharyngeal membrane, cardiogenic areas, and septum transversum are carried into their ventral positions. The cloacal membrane, allantois and connecting stalk are also carried ventrally into position.

12. HEAD AND TAIL FOLDS

STAGE 8

amniotic cavity

(dR)

(dR)

chorionic villus (o)

yolk sac

(o)

allantoic diverticulum

STAGE 8

(dR)

(dB)

(dB)

neural fold

(dR)

(o)

STAGE 10

head fold

amniotic cavity

(o)

tail fold

(o)

(dR)

(dR)

yolk sac

septum transversum

allantois

(o)

STAGE 10

amniotic cavity

neural tube

(o)

(dB)

(o)

(dB)

(o)

STAGE 11

(o)

midgut

amniotic cavity

hindgut

(dR)

(o)

(dR)

foregut

yolk sac

allantois

(o)

STAGE 11

(o)

midgut

intraembryonic coelom

(dB)

(o)

(dB)

communication between intra- and extraembryonic coelom

yolk sac

(o)

amniotic cavity

STAGE 12

(o)

(o)

(dR)

yolk sac

(o)

(dR)

allantois

43

PLACENTA AND FETAL MEMBRANES

13. Derivatives of the Germ Layers: Ectoderm, Mesoderm and Endoderm

All of the tissues of the body develop from three basic germ layers: ectoderm, mesoderm and endoderm. A specialised region of ectoderm called the neuroectoderm also gives rise to numerous tissues.

Most tissues are composed of combinations of the germ layers. If one germ layer causes the cells of another layer to become specialised or differentiate to form specific organs or tissues, the process is called 'induction'.

PLACENTA AND FETAL MEMBRANES

13. DERIVATIVES OF THE GERM LAYERS: ECTODERM, MESODERM, AND ENDODERM

SURFACE ECTODERM (o)

epidermis
hair and nails
cutaneous glands
mammary glands
enamel of teeth
anterior
  pituitary gland
inner ear
lens

NEUROECTODERM (Y)

NEURAL TUBE
  central
    nervous system
  retina
  pineal body
  posterior
    pituitary gland

NEURAL CREST
  cranial and
    sensory ganglia
    and nerves
  adrenal
    medulla
  pigment cells
  part of branchial arch cartilages

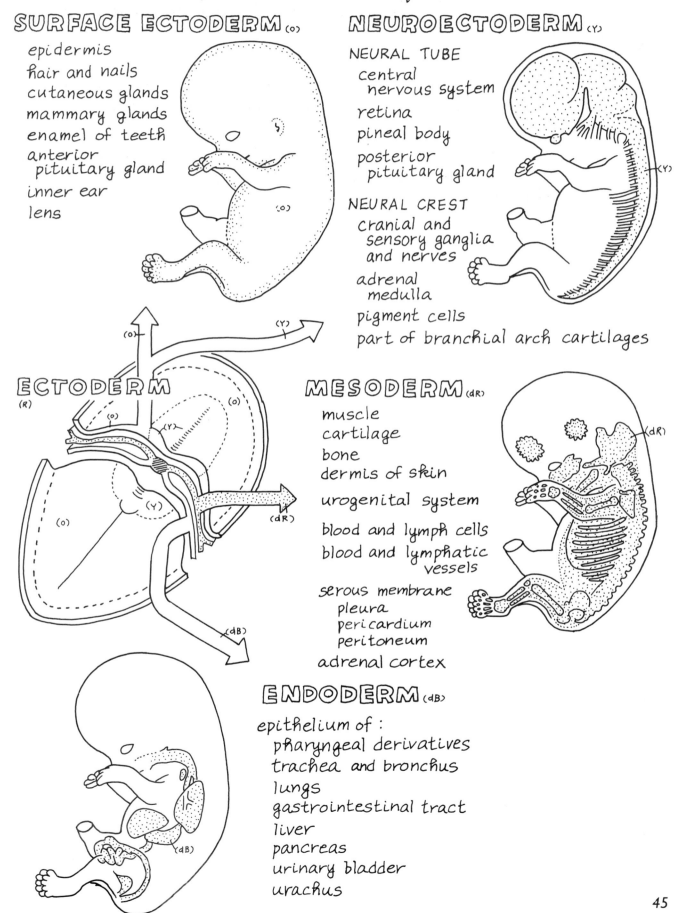

ECTODERM (R)

MESODERM (dR)

muscle
cartilage
bone
dermis of skin
urogenital system
blood and lymph cells
blood and lymphatic
  vessels
serous membrane
  pleura
  pericardium
  peritoneum
adrenal cortex

ENDODERM (dB)

epithelium of:
  pharyngeal derivatives
  trachea and bronchus
  lungs
  gastrointestinal tract
  liver
  pancreas
  urinary bladder
  urachus

The mesoderm layer has many derivatives which are based upon the somite stage of the embryo (for clarity see 11. Somites).

The mesoderm is divided into three main regions; paraxial, intermediate and lateral mesoderm. Each of these three divisions has numerous derivatives, e.g. paraxial mesoderm forms somites. Each somite subdivides into three areas; the dermatome, myotome and sclerotome.

DERIVATIVES OF THE GERM LAYERS: MESODERM AT THE SOMITE STAGE

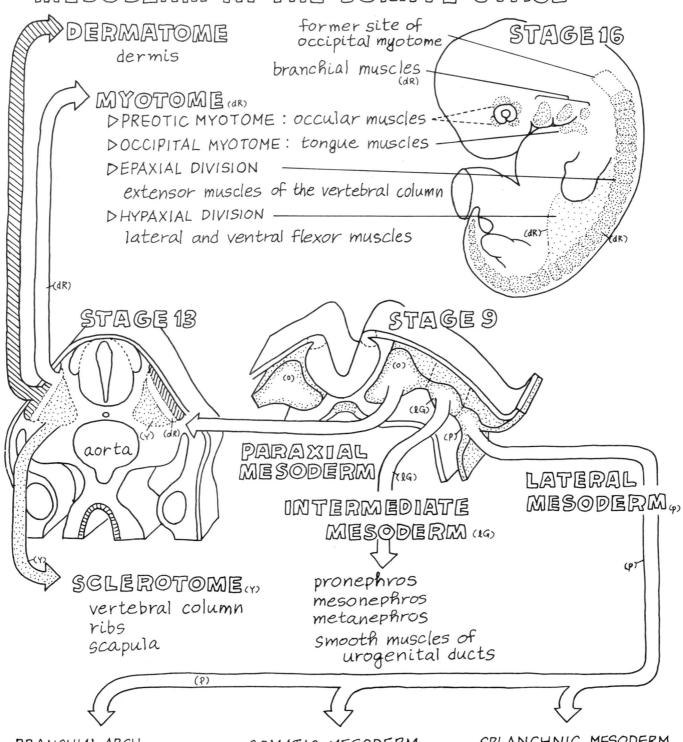

DERMATOME

dermis

former site of occipital myotome

STAGE 16

branchial muscles (dR)

MYOTOME (dR)
▷ PREOTIC MYOTOME : occular muscles
▷ OCCIPITAL MYOTOME : tongue muscles
▷ EPAXIAL DIVISION
  extensor muscles of the vertebral column
▷ HYPAXIAL DIVISION
  lateral and ventral flexor muscles

(dR)

(dR) (dR)

STAGE 13

STAGE 9

(o) (o)

(lG)

aorta (Y) (dR)

(P)

PARAXIAL MESODERM (lG)

LATERAL MESODERM (p)

INTERMEDIATE MESODERM (lG)

(Y)

(P)

SCLEROTOME (Y)

vertebral column
ribs
scapula

pronephros
mesonephros
metanephros
smooth muscles of
  urogenital ducts

(P)

BRANCHIAL ARCH
MESODERM

branchial muscles

· muscles of
   mastication
· facial muscles
· stylopharyngeus muscle
· pharyngolaryngeal muscles

SOMATIC MESODERM

limb muscles
urogenital sphincters
diaphragm muscles
parietal part of
  serous membrane

SPLANCHNIC MESODERM

cardiac muscle
most of smooth muscles

visceral part of
  serous membrane

14. Yolk Sac and Allantois

Extraembryonic Coelom

The cytotrophoblast continues to proliferate and forms a layer of extraembryonic mesoderm separating the amnion and primary yolk sac from the surrounding cytotrophoblast. Spaces then appear in the extraembryonic mesoderm and they fuse to form a larger space, the extraembryonic coelom. The mesoderm is split by this coelom into two layers: the somatic mesoderm, and the splanchnic mesoderm. Later, this coelom becomes the chorionic sac.

Connecting Stalk

The coelom expands until a thick connecting stalk of extraembryonic mesoderm attaches the embryo to the developing placenta. This stalk will later form the umbilical cord.

Secondary Yolk Sac

The primary yolk sac becomes smaller in size as the extraembryonic coelom expands, and a smaller secondary yolk sac forms as hypoblast cells from the embryonic disc grow inside the primary yolk sac. The yolk sac is so named because it is yellow in colour and is involved in early nutrition. Nutrients from the maternal blood diffuse across the extracoelomic membrane, its associated splanchnopleuric mesoderm and into the extraembryonic coelom. They then cross the yolk sac and pass to the embryonic disc.

In Week 3, the yolk sac is also a site for early blood cell and plasma formation. Primordial germ cells also form in the yolk sac walls, and migrate in Week 3 to the site of the future gonads where they will ultimately form the male or female germ cells.

Finally, during Week 4, the dorsal aspect of the yolk sac is incorporated into the embryo to contribute to the respiratory system and primitive gut (epithelium of the lungs, trachea, bronchi and digestive tract).

By Week 10, the small and shrunken yolk sac is attached to the midgut by a narrow yolk stalk. Eventually this stalk will detach from the midgut during its rotation (see **78**. Midgut: Rotation).

Allantois

The allantois is a diverticulum from the secondary yolk sac which grows into the connecting stalk at about Day 16. It, together with the yolk sac, contributes to early blood cell formation during Weeks 3–5. The blood vessels supplying the allantois become the two umbilical veins and the two umbilical arteries.

Later in development, the allantois becomes continuous with the urinary bladder. It eventually may make a small contribution to the apex of the bladder, but the majority of the allantois becomes an involuted tube, the urachus. The urachus finally forms the fibrous median umbilical ligament which is continuous with the umbilicus in the adult.

If the lumen of the allantois remains patent, an urachal cyst, fistula or sinus may form.

14. YOLK SAC AND ALLANTOIS

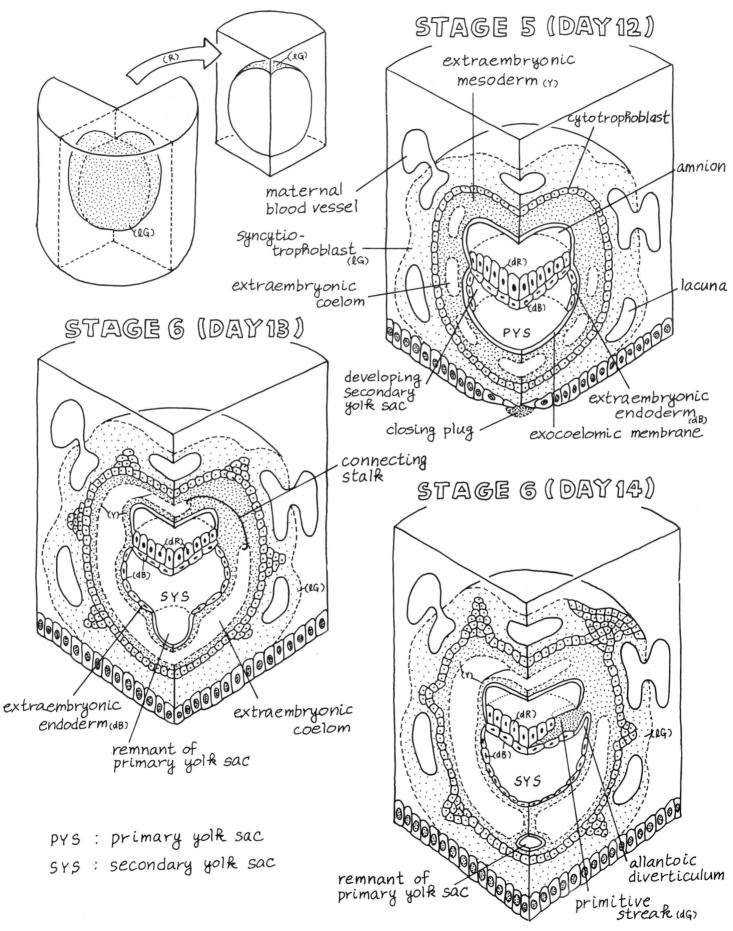

STAGE 5 (DAY 12)

extraembryonic mesoderm (Y)

cytotrophoblast

amnion

maternal blood vessel

syncytio-trophoblast (ℓG)

lacuna

extraembryonic coelom

(dR)

(dB)

PYS

developing secondary yolk sac

extraembryonic endoderm (dB)

closing plug

exocoelomic membrane

STAGE 6 (DAY 13)

connecting stalk

(Y)

(dR)

(dB)

SYS

(ℓG)

extraembryonic endoderm (dB)

extraembryonic coelom

remnant of primary yolk sac

STAGE 6 (DAY 14)

(dR)

(Y)

(dB)

SYS

(ℓG)

remnant of primary yolk sac

allantoic diverticulum

primitive streak (dG)

PYS : primary yolk sac

SYS : secondary yolk sac

15. Amniotic Sac and Chorion

Amniotic Sac

The amniotic cavity forms between the epiblast layer and the overlying cytotrophoblast layer. Cells of the cytotrophoblast form the roof or amnion of the amniotic cavity. The amnion is continuous with the edges of the epiblast layer at its periphery.

Later in development the amnion fuses with the chorion to form the amniochorionic membrane. The amniotic sac is filled with amniotic fluid which completely surrounds the embryo and fetus.

Amniotic fluid has four functions: to act as a cushion to protect the infant; to allow embryonic and fetal movements and to prevent tissue adhesions; to allow symmetrical growth; and to maintain a constant temperature, and to act as a reservoir for fetal metabolites before their excretion by the maternal system. Some amniotic fluid may initially be produced by the amniotic cells, but the majority of the fluid crosses the amnion from the maternal circulation.

The fetus regularly swallows amniotic fluid which is absorbed by the digestive tract. The fetus also produces urine which is passed into the surrounding amniotic fluid.

The composition of the amniotic fluid is maintained by the exchange of large volumes of fluid between the fetal and maternal circulations. This occurs primarily across the placental membrane.

One of the first signs of impending birth is the rupturing of the sac with the escape of amniotic fluid. This is commonly called the 'breaking of the waters.' The amniochorionic membrane is expelled in the third stage of labour along with the placenta and umbilical cord. Amniocentesis is a procedure for withdrawing amniotic fluid, and is commonly done around Week 16. The level of alphafetoprotein in the fluid may be measured; elevated values indicate the presence of a neural tube defect. The cells in the amniotic fluid may also be cultured for the diagnosis of genetic defects.

15. AMNIOTIC SAC AND CHORION

STAGE 6 (sagittal section)

STAGE 6

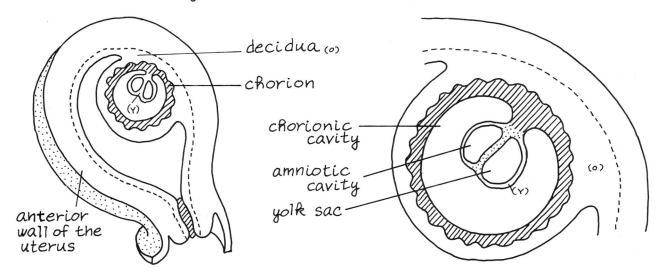

decidua (0)

chorion

chorionic cavity

amniotic cavity

yolk sac

anterior wall of the uterus

PRIMARY VILLUS

SECONDARY VILLUS

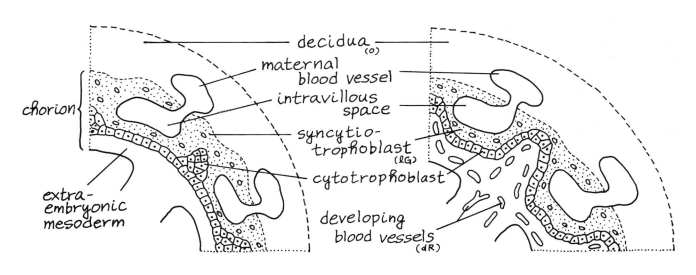

decidua (0)

maternal blood vessel

intravillous space

syncytio-trophoblast (lG)

cytotrophoblast

developing blood vessels (dR)

chorion

extra-embryonic mesoderm

TERTIARY VILLUS

STAGE 9

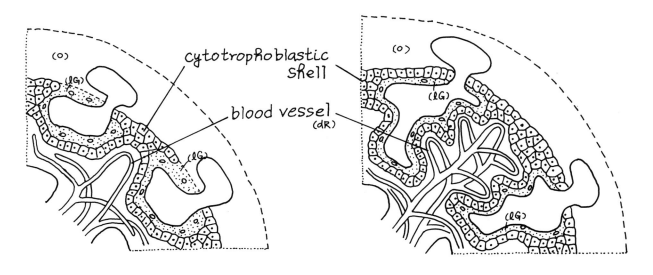

cytotrophoblastic shell

blood vessel (dR)

(0)

(lG)

Chorion

The extraembryonic coelom in the Stage 5 embryo completely surrounds the amniotic sac and yolk sac, except in the region of the connecting stalk (see **14**. Yolk Sac and Allantois).

The layer of extraembryonic somatic mesoderm together with the two layers of trophoblast form the chorion. The extraembryonic coelom is now called the chorionic cavity within the chorionic sac. The embryo, its yolk sac and amniotic cavity are suspended by the connecting stalk within the chorionic cavity.

As the chorionic sac expands in Week 2, the first primary chorionic villi appear on its external surface. These are projections of cytotrophoblast into the syncytiotrophoblast. As soon as the primary villi begin to form they branch.

The secondary chorionic villi form when mesenchyme grows into the primary villi and forms a core. The tertiary chorionic villi develop when some of the mesenchymal core differentiates into blood capillaries which form an artery–capillary–venous network. The cytotrophoblast cells of the tertiary villi extend further into the syncytiotrophoblast layer to form the cytotrophoblastic shell. There are two types of villi. The first are stem or anchoring which attach the chorionic sac to the cytotrophoblastic shell and maternal tissues; the main exchange of metabolic products and gases occurs in the stem villi. The second type of villi are branch villi which grow from the sides of the stem villi.

The artery–capillary–venous network soon forms connections with blood vessels passing into the connecting stalk which are continuous with the embryonic cardiovascular system. At the same time, they also link up with vessels forming in the chorion. By the end of Week 3, embryonic blood is flowing through this network of blood vessels. Nutrients and oxygen diffuse from the maternal blood in the intervillous spaces and pass across the villi into the embryonic blood. Waste products and carbon dioxide diffuse in the opposite direction.

The chorion may be used in chorionic villus biopsy to detect genetic disorders. This should be performed no earlier than 10 weeks. Limb and facial defects have been associated with its use before this age.

Anomalies of the Amniotic Sac and Chorion

Excessive amniotic fluid (polyhydramnios) or a deficiency of amniotic fluid (oligohydramnios) may be associated with fetal abnormalities (e.g. of the palate or urinary system).

Very rarely, a non-invasive tumour (hydatidiform mole) or a highly malignant one (chorionepithelioma) may develop from the chorionic epithelium.

STAGE 12

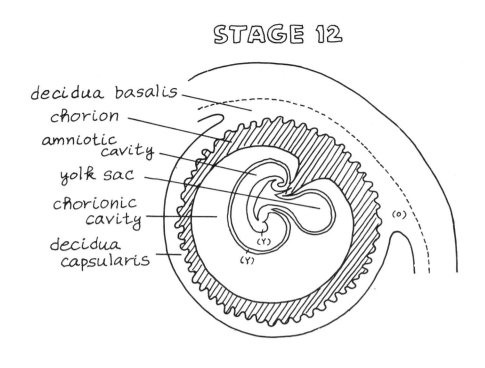

decidua basalis
chorion
amniotic cavity
yolk sac
chorionic cavity
decidua capsularis

(o)
(Y)
(Y)

STAGE 16

STAGE 23

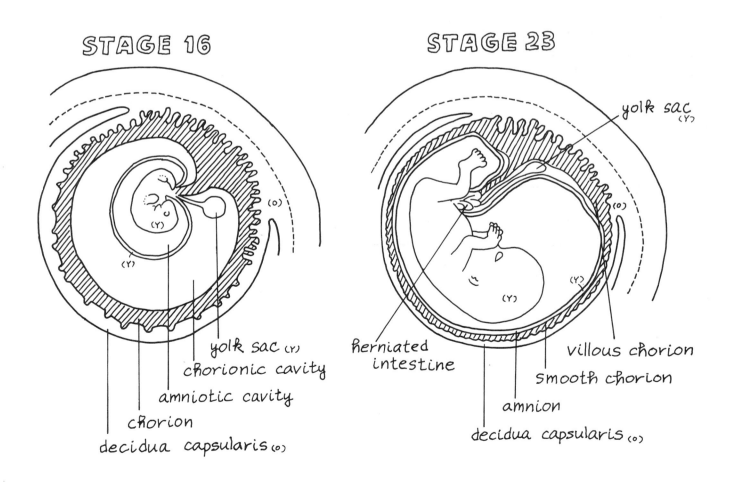

(o)
(Y)
(Y)

yolk sac (Y)
chorionic cavity
amniotic cavity
chorion
decidua capsularis (o)

yolk sac (Y)
(o)
(Y)

herniated intestine
villous chorion
smooth chorion
amnion
decidua capsularis (o)

16. Placental Circulation

The maternal and embryonic (or fetal) circulations remain largely separated by the placental membrane. Up to the sixth month, this membrane consists of four fetal layers: fetal capillary endothelium; connective tissue in the villus; cytotrophoblast; and syncytiotrophoblast. Most substances are able to pass from the maternal to the fetal circulation through this membrane, but some molecules may be excluded.

Later in fetal development, three changes occur: the placental membrane thins; nuclear aggregations in the syncytiotrophoblast (syncytial knots) break free and enter the maternal circulation; and fibrinoid material forms on the villi.

Maternal and Fetal Circulation

Maternal blood in the spiral arteries enters the intervillous space through gaps in the cytotrophoblastic shell, and bathes the villi. This blood is rich in oxygen and nutrients. The embryonic blood is delivered to the placenta via the two umbilical arteries which branch on the chorionic plate to form chorionic vessels supplying the chorionic villi. This blood is deoxygenated and contains metabolic and gaseous wastes. The exchange of nutrients, wastes and gases occurs across the villi between the maternal and embryonic blood. The maternal blood then leaves via an endometrial vein, while the embryonic blood returns to the embryo via veins which join to form the umbilical vein.

Placental Functions

There are four main functions of the placenta. The first is to transport materials and gases to and from the embryonic and maternal circulations. This includes the diffusion of oxygen from the maternal blood into the embryonic blood and the diffusion of carbon dioxide in the opposite direction. Nutrients (water, inorganic salts, vitamins, fats, proteins, and carbohydrates) also pass from the maternal circulation to the fetal one. The fetal waste products diffuse into the maternal blood.

The second placental function is to produce hormones (oestrogens, progesterone, human chorionic somatomammotropin, and human chorionic gonadotropin).

The third function is to store and release carbohydrates, proteins, iron and calcium as required by the fetus.

The fourth function is to prevent microorganisms from crossing the placental membrane to the fetus. Most bacteria are unable to cross, but this is not true of certain viruses.

16. PLACENTAL CIRCULATION

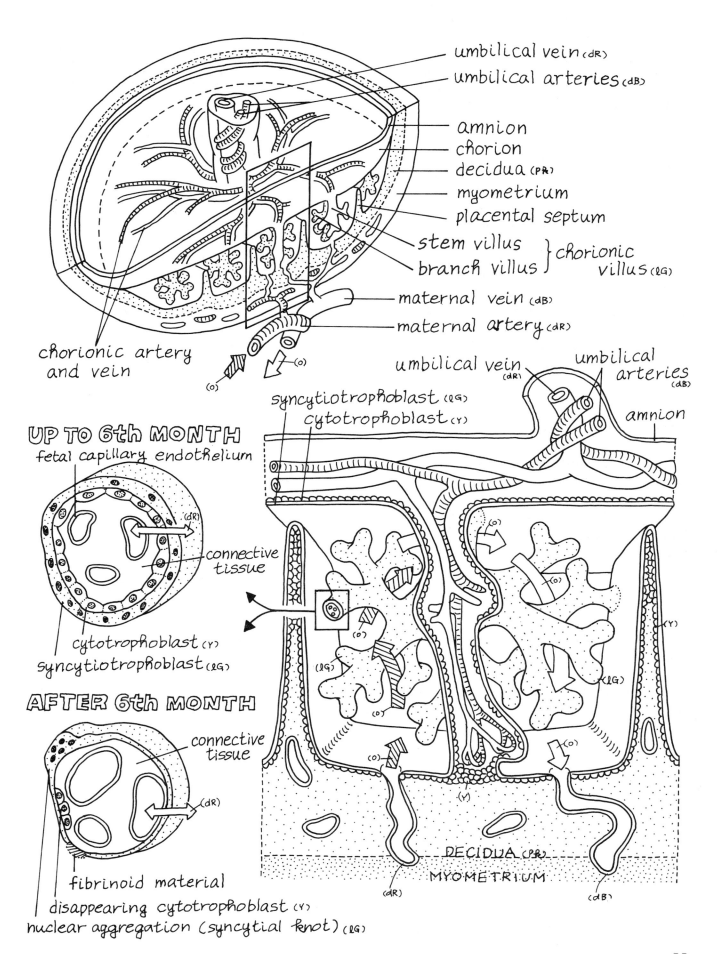

umbilical vein (dR)

umbilical arteries (dB)

amnion

chorion

decidua (PR)

myometrium

placental septum

stem villus

branch villus } chorionic villus (LG)

maternal vein (dB)

maternal artery (dR)

chorionic artery and vein

syncytiotrophoblast (LG)

cytotrophoblast (Y)

umbilical vein (dR)

umbilical arteries (dB)

amnion

UP TO 6th MONTH

fetal capillary endothelium

connective tissue

(dR)

cytotrophoblast (Y)

syncytiotrophoblast (LG)

AFTER 6th MONTH

connective tissue

(dR)

fibrinoid material

disappearing cytotrophoblast (Y)

nuclear aggregation (syncytial knot) (LG)

DECIDUA (PR)

MYOMETRIUM

(dR)

(dB)

55

17. Multiple Pregnancy

The most common naturally occurring multiple birth is twins. These are either fraternal (dizygotic) twins derived from two oocytes, or identical (monozygotic) twins derived from a single oocyte.

Each dizygotic twin has an amnion, a chorion, and a placenta which may or may not be fused with that of its twin.

A monozygotic twin commonly has its own amnion, but a shared chorion and a shared placenta. Some, however, also share one amnion if the twins formed after the amniotic cavity had formed.

Triplets, quadruplets etc. are derived from one or more oocytes. Superovulation may be induced clinically by the use of drugs to treat infertility. Multiple births usually result in premature deliveries.

Anomalies of Multiple Conceptions

Conjoint twins are formed if the inner cell mass or embryonic disc does not completely divide during twinning.

17. MULTIPLE PREGNANCY

▷ DIZYGOTIC TWINS ◁

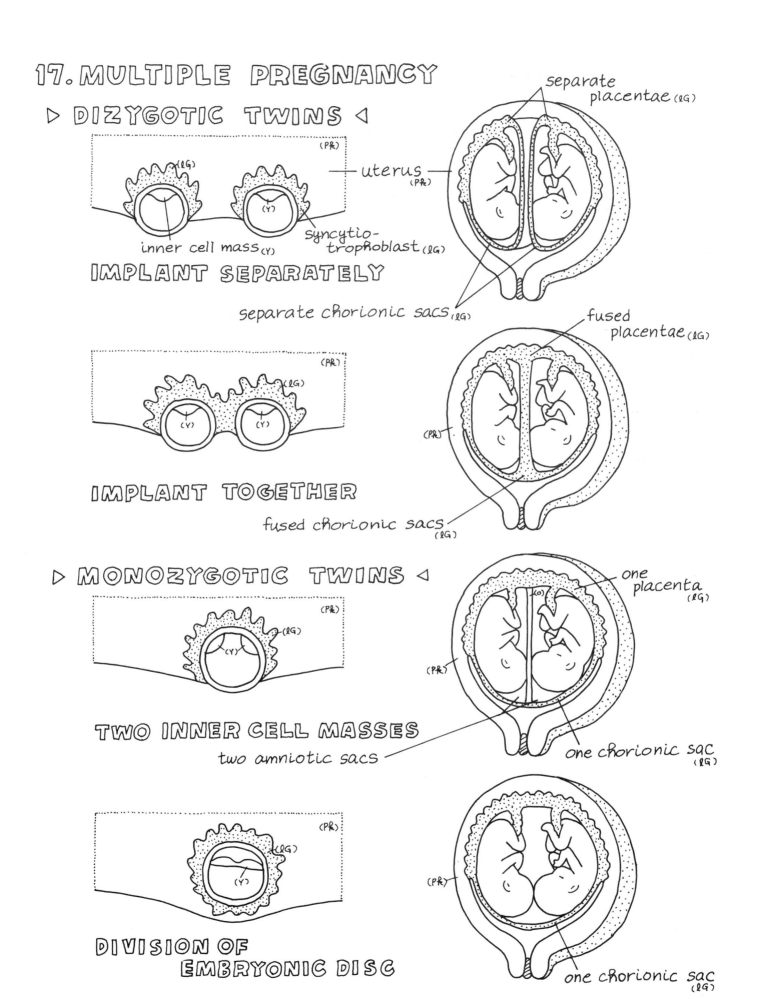

separate
placentae (ℓG)

(ℓG)

(PK)

uterus (PK)

inner cell mass (Y)

syncytio-
trophoblast (ℓG)

IMPLANT SEPARATELY

separate chorionic sacs (ℓG)

(PK)

(Y)   (Y)

(ℓG)

fused
placentae (ℓG)

(PK)

IMPLANT TOGETHER

fused chorionic sacs (ℓG)

▷ MONOZYGOTIC TWINS ◁

(PK)

(ℓG)

(Y)

one
placenta (ℓG)

(O)

(PK)

TWO INNER CELL MASSES

two amniotic sacs

one chorionic sac (ℓG)

(PK)

(ℓG)

(Y)

(PK)

**DIVISION OF
EMBRYONIC DISC**

one chorionic sac (ℓG)

18. Full Term Placenta

The full term placenta has two parts: maternal and fetal.

The maternal part is derived from the decidua basalis, and its surface is composed of approximately 10–38 cotyledons. Each cotyledon has a main stem villus and its branches. The surface of the maternal part is covered by a thin layer of decidua basalis.

The fetal part forms from the villous chorion and is covered with a smooth layer of amnion which also covers the umbilical cord near its centre. The umbilical blood vessels are visible through the amnion radiating from the cord. As the vessels sub-divide on the surface, they form the chorionic vessels supplying the chorionic villi. The layer of amnion is continuous with the amniotic and chorionic sac.

The maternal and fetal parts are joined by anchoring villi and the cytotrophoblastic shell.

The average full-term umbilical cord is approximately the same length as the fetus (55 cm long) with as many as 40 twists. It contains two arteries carrying deoxygenated blood and one vein carrying oxygenated blood surrounded by a loose, connective tissue called Wharton's jelly. Following the delivery of the infant, the placenta, fetal membranes and umbilical cord are delivered as the 'afterbirth', during the third stage of labour or parturition. The placenta is flattened and discoid in shape, and weighs approximately 500–600g.

Anomalies of the Umbilical Cord

Abnormally short or long umbilical cords or a single umbilical artery may be associated with fetal abnormalities.

18. FULL TERM PLACENTA

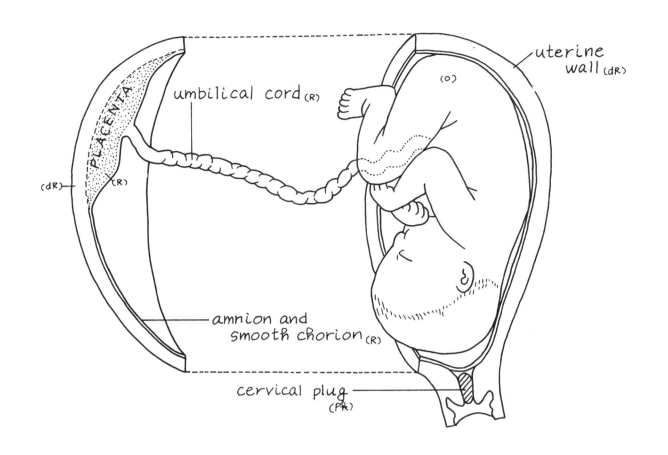

PLACENTA

umbilical cord (R)

uterine wall (dR)

(O)

(dR)

(R)

amnion and smooth chorion (R)

cervical plug (PR)

MATERNAL SURFACE

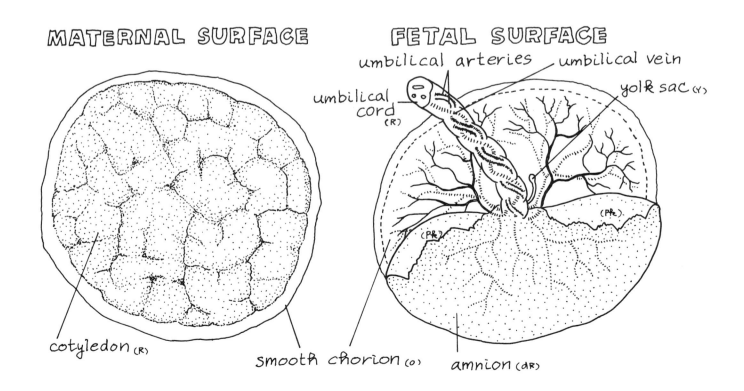

cotyledon (R)

smooth chorion (O)

FETAL SURFACE

umbilical arteries

umbilical vein

umbilical cord (R)

yolk sac (Y)

(PR)

(PR)

amnion (dR)

19. Parturition

The delivery or parturition of a full term infant occurs after a gestation of 266 days, i.e. approximately 38 weeks after fertilisation. There are three stages of childbirth or labour: the first stage ends at the complete dilatation of the cervix; the second stage is the delivery of the baby; and the third stage is the delivery of the placenta, fetal membranes and umbilical cord.

The first stage of labour occurs when there are regular contractions of the uterus, and ends with the complete dilatation of the cervix. This stage lasts approximately 10–12 hours for first pregnancies (primigravidas) or less than 7 hours for multigravidas (or multiparous) women who have previously delivered infants.

The second stage ends with the delivery of the baby. Primigravidas usually average 50 minutes in the second stage of labour, while multigravidas average 20 minutes.

The third stage of labour ends when the afterbirth, consisting of the placenta and its associated membranes, is expelled. This stage is usually less than 10 minutes.

The placenta separates through the decidua basalis. The decidua basalis is later sloughed off with further uterine bleeding. The maternal spiral arteries at the placental site constrict as the muscles of the myometrium contract and excessive blood loss is prevented.

Anomalies of Parturition

The normal position for delivery of the infant is by cephalic presentation. Other positions, such as breech presentation, usually impede and lengthen the delivery.

19. PARTURITION

FIRST STAGE : DILATATION OF THE CERVIX

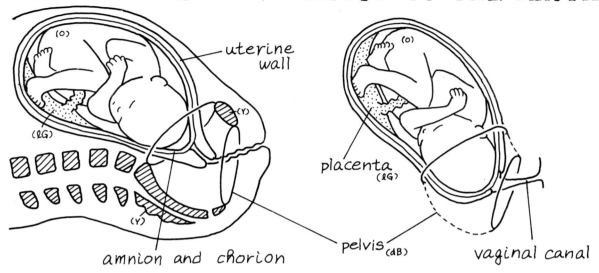

uterine wall

(o)

(ℓG)

(Y)

placenta (ℓG)

amnion and chorion

pelvis (dB)

vaginal canal

SECOND STAGE : DELIVERY OF THE BABY

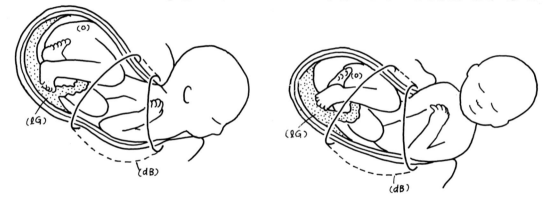

(o)

(ℓG)

(dB)

(ℓG)

(o)

(dB)

THIRD STAGE : DELIVERY OF THE PLACENTA

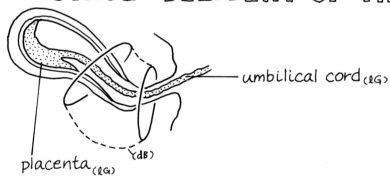

umbilical cord (ℓG)

placenta (ℓG)

(dB)

DURATION OF EACH STAGE

STAGE	PRIMIGRAVIDAS	MULTIGRAVIDAS
1	10 - 12 HOURS	< 7 HOURS
2	30 - 90 MINS	< 20 MINS
3	5 - 25 MINS	5 - 25 MINS

CARDIOVASCULAR SYSTEM

20. Blood and Lymphatic Formation

Blood Formation

Groups of mesenchyme cells condense to form blood islands (see **21.** Early Blood Vessels and Aortic Arches). Those cells in the centre of the blood islands form nucleated blood cells and plasma. Up to Week 4, the only blood cells are red blood cells. Blood formation begins in Week 5 in the embryonic yolk sac, and at Week 6 it begins in the liver. Later, blood also forms in the spleen (2.5 months), and in the bone marrow (2–3 months). By 2.5 months the liver produces coagulation factors. Fetal blood is nucleated until the third month. Lymphocytes also arise from primitive stem cells in the yolk sac mesenchyme. Later, they arise from the liver and spleen and invade the bone marrow to form lymphoblasts.

By birth, blood formation has ceased in the liver and spleen and haemopoiesis occurs in the red marrow of all the bones of the skeleton. Fetal haemoglobin predominates at birth.

Lymphatic Formation

Lymphatic vessels develop in Weeks 5–6 in a similar way to the formation of blood vessels. The early vessels join together to form a closed network of lymphatics and lymph sacs. There are six primary lymph sacs (two jugular, two iliac, one retroperitoneal, and one is the cisterna chyli). Vessels from these sacs pass primarily along main veins.

Lymph nodes form during the fetal period when the sacs (except the superior portion of the cisterna chyli) are transformed. Some mesenchyme cells migrate into the sacs and break them up into lymph sinuses. Other mesenchyme cells give rise to the connective tissue and capsule. Lymphocytes in the early lymph nodes arise from the thymus gland; later, some mesenchyme cells differentiate in the nodes to form lymphocytes. Lymph nodules are present at birth.

CARDIOVASCULAR SYSTEM

20. BLOOD AND LYMPHATIC FORMATION

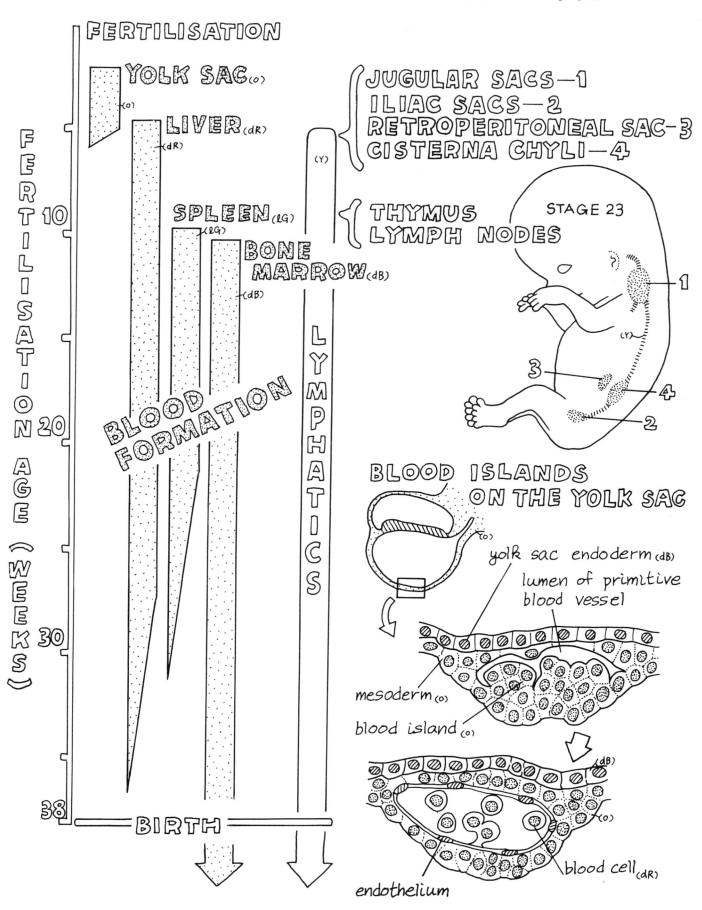

FERTILISATION

YOLK SAC (o)

(o)

LIVER (dR)

(dR)

JUGULAR SACS—1
ILIAC SACS—2
RETROPERITONEAL SAC—3
CISTERNA CHYLI—4

(Y)

SPLEEN (lG)

(lG)

THYMUS
LYMPH NODES

BONE
MARROW (dB)

(dB)

FERTILISATION AGE (WEEKS)

10

20

30

38

BLOOD
FORMATION

LYMPHATICS

BIRTH

STAGE 23

1

(Y)

3

4

2

BLOOD ISLANDS
ON THE YOLK SAC

(o)

yolk sac endoderm (dB)
lumen of primitive
blood vessel

mesoderm (o)

blood island (o)

(dB)

(o)

blood cell (dR)

endothelium

63

21. Early Blood Vessels and Aortic Arches

Early Blood Vessels

Blood vessels are derived from groups of mesenchyme cells (angioblasts) which are termed blood islands. Those cells in the centre of the island will form the primitive blood cells; those on the periphery will form the blood vessel endothelium. The blood islands link up to form blood vessels. The heart develops in the cardiogenic area of mesenchyme located in front of the primitive knot; during head fold formation this area is carried ventrally into the midline. There, paired endocardial heart tubes form, and they fuse in the midline to form the primitive heart tube.

Early blood vessels form on the yolk sac (vitelline vessels), in the embryo (cardinal vessels), and in the connecting stalk and chorion (umbilical and chorionic vessels). These vessels link the early cardiovascular system in the embryo with the yolk sac vessels and the extraembryonic vessels of the connecting stalk, chorion and placenta.

All of the vitelline, cardinal and umbilical vessels are paired, as well as, the two dorsal aortae. One vitelline vein, one cardinal vein and one umbilical vein on each side of the early embryo's body deliver blood to the heart. Oxygenated blood from the placenta is carried to the embryo's heart via the two umbilical veins and deoxygenated blood is returned to the placenta via the two umbilical arteries. Blood from the yolk sac is carried to the embryo via the vitelline veins to the early heart and that from the embryo's tissues is carried via the cardinal veins. The names of the cardinal veins are determined by the parts of the body they drain. The head region is drained by the anterior cardinals and the body region by the posterior cardinals. The anterior and posterior cardinals join to form the common cardinal vein on each side to enter the heart. (See **84**. Kidneys: Mesonephros, for an explanation of the relationship between the cardinal system and the second stage of kidney development.)

The two dorsal aortae fuse caudally to the branchial arches to form a single vessel.

21. EARLY BLOOD VESSELS AND AORTIC ARCHES
STAGE 8

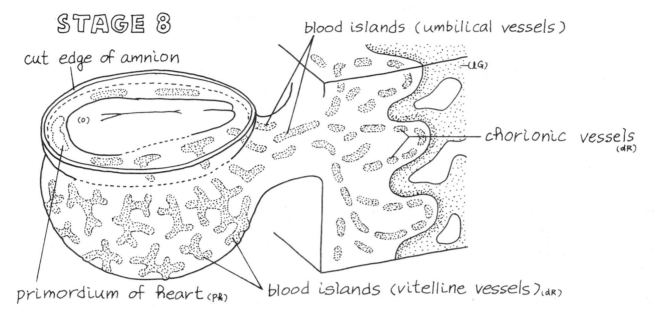

blood islands (umbilical vessels)

(1G)

cut edge of amnion

(0)

chorionic vessels (dR)

primordium of heart (PR)

blood islands (vitelline vessels) (dR)

STAGE 11

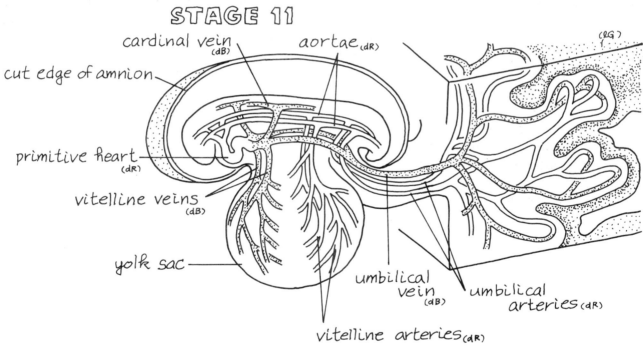

cardinal vein (dB)

aortae (dR)

(lG)

cut edge of amnion

primitive heart (dR)

vitelline veins (dB)

yolk sac

umbilical vein (dB)

umbilical arteries (dR)

vitelline arteries (dR)

Aortic Arches

Blood vessels arise from the aortic sac to supply each branchial arch. The fifth arch and its artery are often rudimentary or absent.

The first and second arch arteries will largely disappear. The third arch arteries become the common carotid arteries and the proximal part of the internal carotid arteries.

The fourth arch arteries persist but form different vessels on each side of the body. The right fourth aortic arch forms the proximal part of the right subclavian artery. On the left, it forms part of the arch of the aorta.

The fifth arch has no derivatives.

The sixth arch arteries persist but form different vessels on each side of the body. The right sixth aortic arch becomes the right pulmonary artery. The left sixth aortic arch forms the left pulmonary artery and the ductus arteriosus.

The ductus arteriosus is a vessel connecting the pulmonary trunk and the aorta. Blood shunted through this vessel bypasses the lungs which are non-inflated.

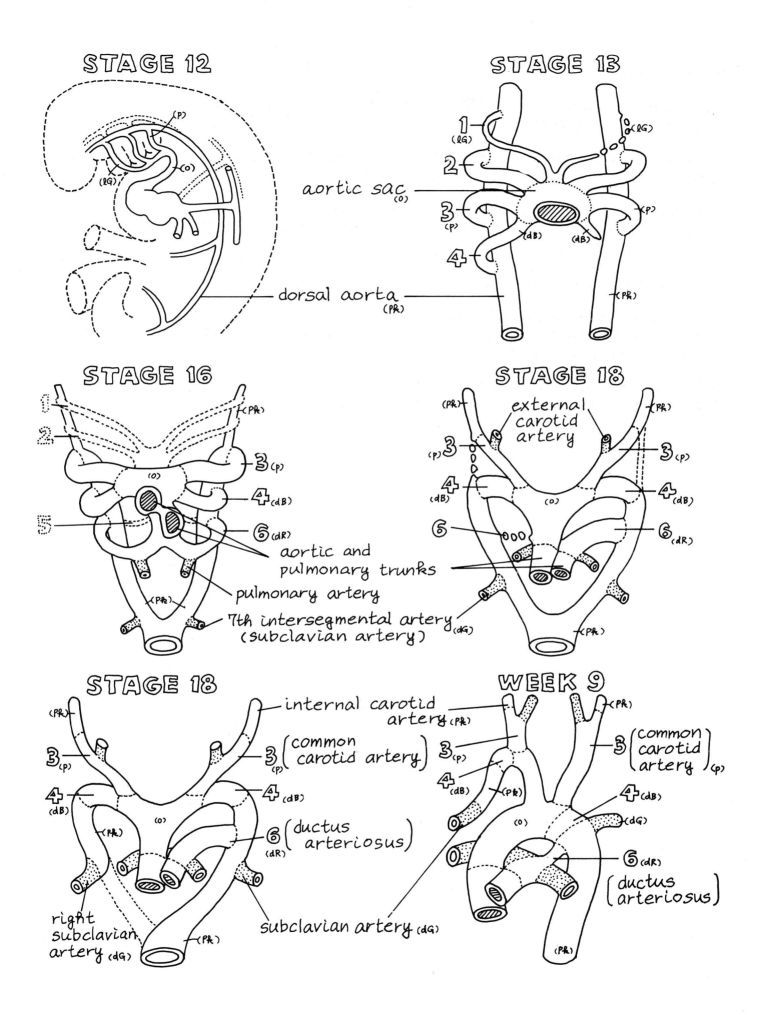

STAGE 12

(P)
(ℓG)
(O)

dorsal aorta
(PR)

STAGE 13

1 (ℓG)
2
3 (P)
4
(ℓG)
(P)
(dB) (dB)
(PR)

aortic sac (O)

dorsal aorta (PR)

STAGE 16

1
2
3 (P)
4 (dB)
5
6 (dR)
(PR)
(O)
(PR)

aortic and pulmonary trunks

pulmonary artery

7th intersegmental artery (subclavian artery) (dG)

STAGE 18

external carotid artery
(PR)
(P) 3
4 (dB)
6
(O)
(PR)
3 (P)
4 (dB)
6 (dR)
(dG)
(PR)

STAGE 18

internal carotid artery (PR)
(PR)
3 (P)
4 (dB)
(PR)
3 (P) (common carotid artery)
4 (dB)
6 (dR) (ductus arteriosus)
right subclavian artery (dG)
(O)
(PR)
subclavian artery (dG)

WEEK 9

(PR)
3 (P)
4 (dB)
(PR)
0
(O)
0
3 (common carotid artery) (P)
4 (dB)
(dG)
6 (dR)
(ductus arteriosus)
(PR)

67

22. Portal Vein Formation

Vitelline and Hepatic Veins

The two vitelline veins pass from the yolk sac to the sinus venosus of the heart. In doing so they go through the mesenchyme of the septum transversum. Then as the liver forms in the septum transversum, it intermingles with the vitelline veins and a network of blood vessels is formed.

The hepatic veins form from the remains of the right vitelline vein.

Umbilical Veins

The two umbilical veins also pass through the septum transversum from the placenta to the sinus venosus. As the liver forms, a connecting branch then develops between each umbilical vein and the vitelline vein network. Once these two new channels have formed, the part of the umbilical vein leading into the sinus venosus disappears. Blood from the left umbilical vein becomes the predominant flow from the placenta and crosses the liver to the developing inferior vena cava in a new channel, the ductus venosus. This channel serves to direct blood from the placenta to the heart.

Portal Vein

The portal vein forms from an anastomotic network of the vitelline veins around the duodenum. That portion of the right vitelline vein nearest the liver disappears.

After Birth

The vestige of the left umbilical vein can be recognised as the fibrous ligamentum teres, and the vestige of the ductus venosus is the ligamentum venosum.

22. PORTAL VEIN FORMATION

STAGE 12

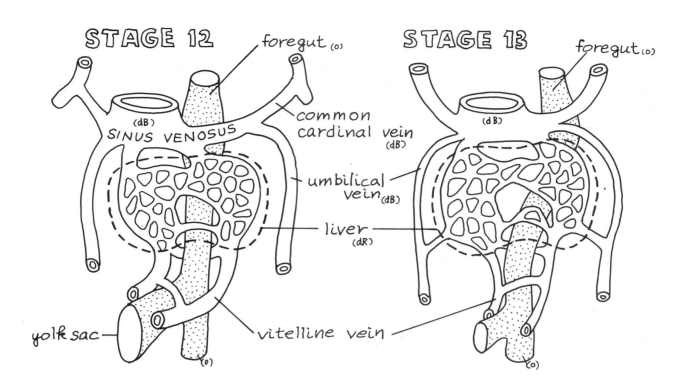

foregut (o)

common
cardinal vein
(dB)

(dB)
SINUS VENOSUS

umbilical
vein (dB)

liver
(dR)

yolk sac

vitelline vein

STAGE 13

foregut (o)

(dB)

STAGE 15

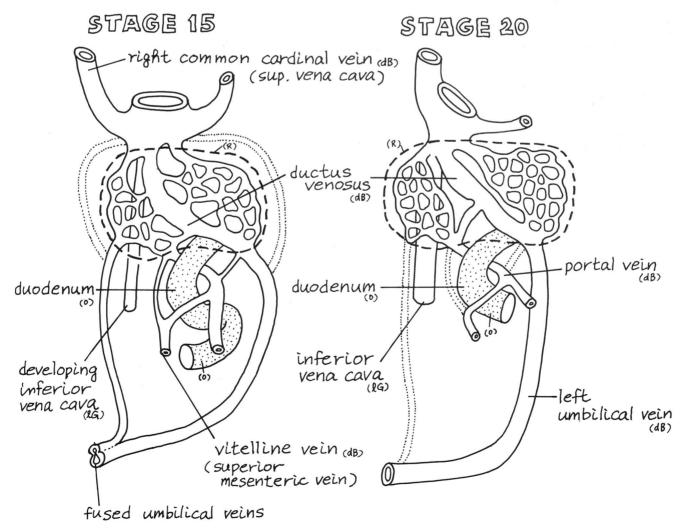

right common cardinal vein (dB)
(sup. vena cava)

(R)

ductus
venosus
(dB)

duodenum
(o)

developing
inferior
vena cava
(lG)

vitelline vein (dB)
(superior
mesenteric vein)

fused umbilical veins

STAGE 20

(R)

portal vein
(dB)

duodenum
(o)

inferior
vena cava
(lG)

left
umbilical vein
(dB)

23. Formation of the Venous System

Two additional sets of veins develop near to the cardinal veins. A ventral network called the subcardinal veins, and a network dorsal to the posterior cardinals called the supracardinal veins.

Inferior Vena Cava

The adult inferior vena cava forms from four primordia:

1. A terminal portion from the right vitelline vein and hepatic vein and sinusoids.
2. A segment cranial to the renal segment which is derived from the right subcardinal veins.
3. A renal segment formed from the anastomosis of the supracardinal and subcardinal veins.
4. A segment caudal to the renal segment formed from the right supracardinal vein.

23. FORMATION OF THE VENOUS SYSTEM

STAGE 13

STAGE 13

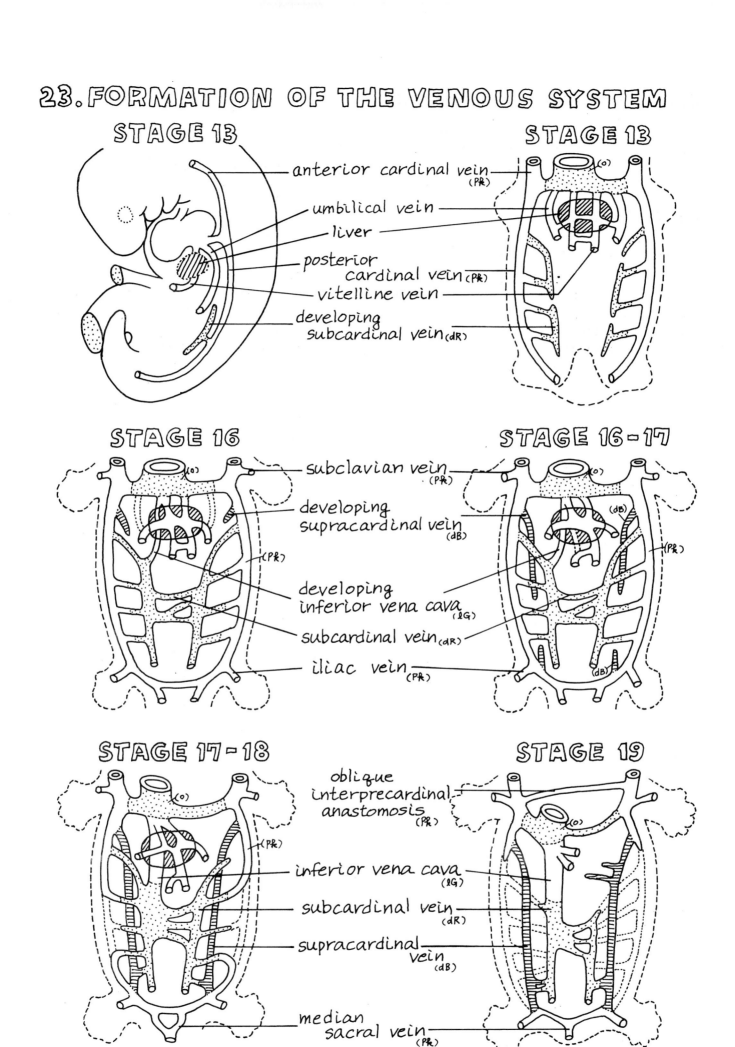

anterior cardinal vein (PR)

umbilical vein

liver

posterior cardinal vein (PR)

vitelline vein

developing subcardinal vein (dR)

STAGE 16

STAGE 16-17

subclavian vein (PR)

developing supracardinal vein (dB)

developing inferior vena cava (lG)

subcardinal vein (dR)

iliac vein (PR)

STAGE 17-18

STAGE 19

oblique interprecardinal anastomosis (PR)

inferior vena cava (lG)

subcardinal vein (dR)

supracardinal vein (dB)

median sacral vein (PR)

Thoracic and Abdominal Veins

The renal veins, gonadal veins and suprarenal veins develop from the supracardinal veins and anastomosis.

The iliac veins are derivatives of the caudal portion of the postcardinal veins.

The hemiazygous vein and azygous vein are derivatives of the supracardinal veins.

The oblique vein of the heart develops from an oblique connecting vessel between the two anterior cardinal veins.

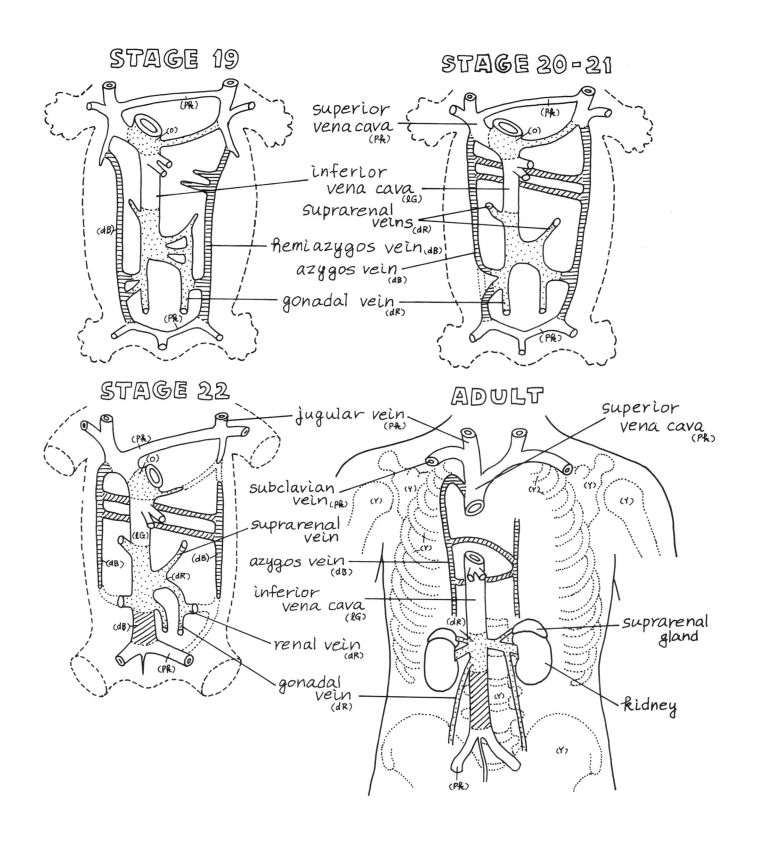

STAGE 19

(PR)
(0)
(dB)
(PR)

STAGE 20-21

superior
vena cava
(PR)

(0)

inferior
vena cava
(LG)

suprarenal
veins (dR)

hemiazygos vein (dB)

azygos vein
(dB)

gonadal vein
(dR)

(PR)

STAGE 22

(PR)
(0)
(LG)
(dB)
(dB)
(dR)
(dB)
(PR)

jugular vein
(PR)

subclavian
vein (PR)

suprarenal
vein

azygos vein
(dB)

inferior
vena cava
(LG)

renal vein
(dR)

gonadal
vein
(dR)

ADULT

superior
vena cava
(PR)

(Y)
(Y)
(Y)
(Y)
(Y)

(dR)

(Y)

(Y)

suprarenal
gland

kidney

(PR)

24. Early Heart Development

Paired endocardial heart tubes form from mesenchymal cardiogenic cords. They then fuse in the midline to form a single heart tube. Splanchnic mesenchyme surrounding this tube will later form the myocardium and epicardium.

Five dilations of the heart tube mark distinct regions, moving from the caudal to the cephalic end of the tube these are: the sinus venosus, the primitive atrium, the primitive ventricle, the bulbus cordis, and the truncus arteriosus. Blood from the umbilical veins, vitelline veins and common cardinal veins on each side of the body enters the sinus venosus and moves cephalically through the heart tube to the truncus arteriosus.

The primitive heart is anchored at both ends; caudally the sinus venosus is partly embedded in the septum transversum (future central tendon of the diaphragm), and cephalically is attached to the aortic sac and its aortic arch arteries. The anchored heart tube grows rapidly, and the elongating tube bends back upon itself to form a 'U' shaped bulboventricular loop. As the bulboventricular loop forms, the primitive atrium is carried *behind* (dorsal to) the primitive ventricle. Both the primitive atrium and ventricle then expand and enlarge to form the two atria and two ventricles.

24. EARLY HEART DEVELOPMENT

STAGE 9

mesenchyme

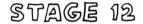

T (dR)
B (Y)
V (O)
A (lG)

STAGE 10

1
AS
(dR)
T
B
(Y)
V
(O)
A (lG)
(dB)
S

STAGE 11

1
AS
2
(dR)
T
B
(Y)
V
(O)
A (lG)
(dB)
S

STAGE 12

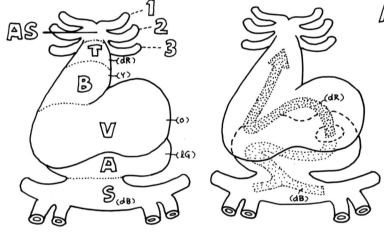

AS
1
2
3
T
(dR)
(Y)
B
V
(O)
(lG)
A
S (dB)
(dR)
(dB)

AS: AORTIC SAC

T: TRUNCUS ARTERIOSUS (dR)

B: BULBUS CORDIS (Y)

A: ATRIUM (lG)

V: VENTRICLE (O)

S: SINUS VENOSUS (dB)

1~6: AORTIC ARCHES

STAGE 12

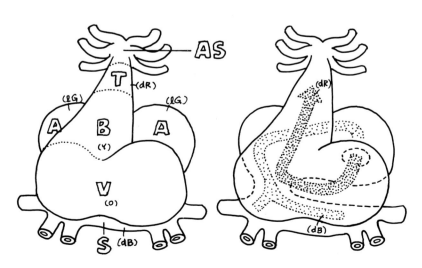

AS
T (dR)
(lG) A
B (Y)
A (lG)
V (O)
S (dB)
(dR)
(dB)

STAGE 16

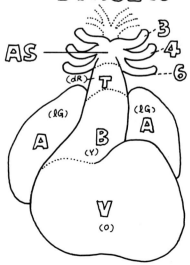

AS
3
4
6
(dR)
T
(lG) A
B (Y)
A (lG)
V (O)

25. Division of the Heart into Four Chambers

During Weeks 4–5, the single heart tube is divided into four chambers: two atria and two ventricles.

The right atrium and ventricle are separated from the left atrium and ventricle by the endocardial cushions. These proliferations of mesenchyme appear on the dorsal and ventral walls in the midline, grow toward one another and fuse. The result is a right and left atrioventricular (AV) canal.

Atria

Two atria form when a membranous sheet, called the septum primum, grows from the dorsal wall and fuses with the endocardial cushion. As it grows, the intervening gap between the wall and the cushion is called the foramen primum. The sheet forms a wall between the two atria. Before the septum primum fuses with the endocardial cushion and closes the foramen primum, an opening appears in the superior wall of the septum primum. This second opening, or foramen secundum, allows blood to flow from the right atrium to the left atrium. Backflow of the blood is prevented by the septum secundum which grows from the ventral wall and to the right of the septum primum. This membranous valve overlaps the foramen secundum which is now called the foramen ovale. The remains of the septum primum now form the valve of the foramen ovale. The inferior border of the septum secundum is called the crista dividens.

The embryonic atrium is identifiable in the adult as the auricle, i.e. those regions of the atrium with roughened walls. In the right atrium, the smooth walls are tissue originating from the incorporated right horn of the sinus venosus. The smooth wall of the left atrium is derived from the incorporated pulmonary vein.

Ventricles

The primitive ventricle is divided into two chambers when a muscular ridge forms in the midline floor and grows towards the endocardial cushion. Later, this ridge will form the muscular part of the interventricular septum. As the interventricular septum slowly grows towards the cushion, the intervening interventricular foramen allows communication between the two ventricles. This opening persists until Week 7, when the foramen closes by the fusion of three membranes: the interventricular septum (membranous), the bulbar ridge, and the aorticopulmonary septum. The area where they fuse is called the membranous part of the interventricular septum.

The right ventricle is primarily formed from the bulbus cordis, while the left ventricle forms from the primitive ventricle. These areas are all identifiable in the adult by their roughened walls. The smooth parts of the right and left ventricles are those regions of the bulbar ridge and aorticopulmonary septum.

25. DIVISION INTO FOUR CHAMBERS

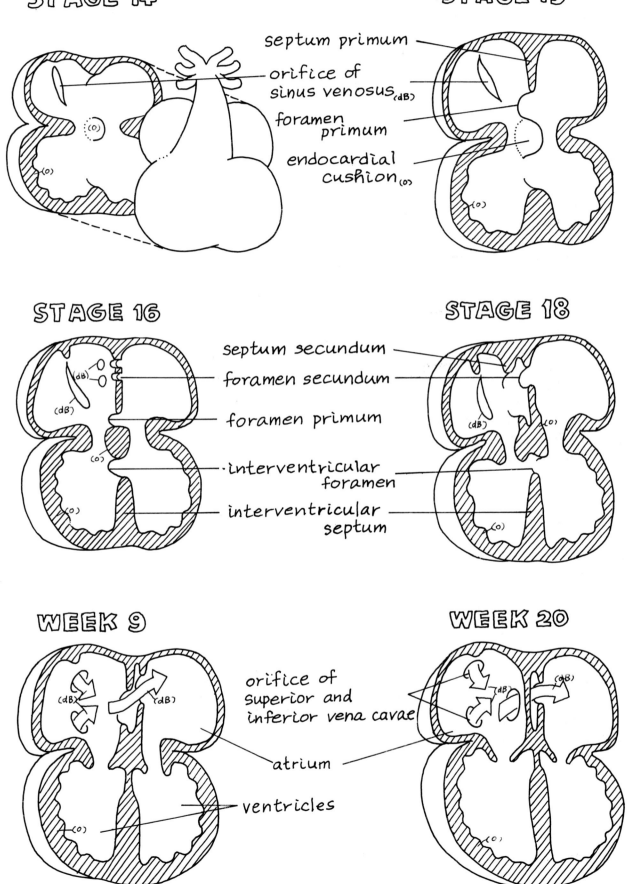

STAGE 14

STAGE 15

septum primum

orifice of
sinus venosus(dB)

foramen
primum

endocardial
cushion(o)

STAGE 16

STAGE 18

septum secundum

foramen secundum

foramen primum

interventricular
foramen

interventricular
septum

WEEK 9

WEEK 20

orifice of
superior and
inferior vena cavae

atrium

ventricles

26. Formation of the Pulmonary and Aortic Trunks

The bulbus cordis and truncus arteriosus are divided longitudinally by a spiral septum into the ascending aorta and pulmonary trunk. The aorticopulmonary septum is formed by two intertwining truncal ridges and bulbar ridges which spiral downwards to form these two main arterial trunks.

Conducting System of the Heart

The sinoatrial node originally forms in the wall of the right horn of the sinus venosus. When the right horn is incorporated in the right atrium, the node is also incorporated.

The atrioventricular node and bundle form from cells in the atrioventricular canal region and sinus venosus.

The sinoatrial node, and the atrioventricular node and bundle become richly innervated.

26. PULMONARY AND AORTIC TRUNK FORMATION

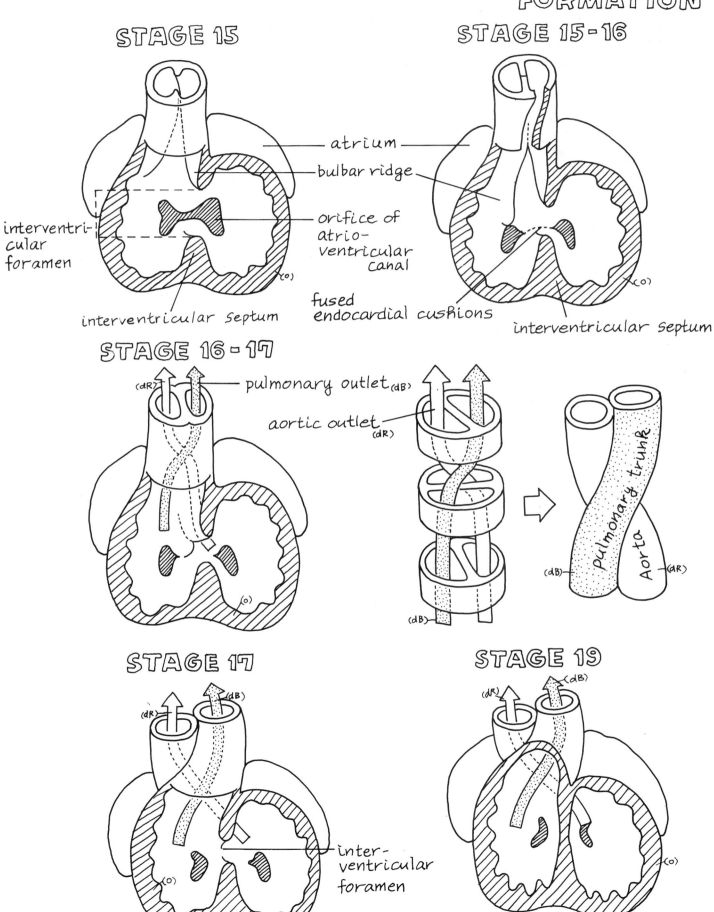

STAGE 15

interventri-
cular
foramen

interventricular septum

atrium

bulbar ridge

orifice of
atrio-
ventricular
canal

STAGE 15-16

fused
endocardial cushions

interventricular septum

STAGE 16-17

pulmonary outlet (dB)

aortic outlet (dR)

(dR)

(dB)

pulmonary trunk

Aorta (dR)

STAGE 17

inter-
ventricular
foramen

STAGE 19

27. Formation of the Vena Cavae and Coronary Sinus

As the bulboventricular loop forms, the primitive atrium is carried behind (dorsal to) the primitive ventricle. The sinus venosus attached to the primitive atrium has a right and a left horn with three vessels entering each horn. The vessels are the common cardinal vein, the vitelline vein, and the umbilical vein.

As the two atria form, the right horn of the sinus venosus which has enlarged is incorporated into the wall of the right atrium. The embryonic atrium persists as the right auricle, the rough-walled appendage of the atrium.

The smaller left horn of the sinus venosus forms the coronary sinus. The right vitelline vein contributes to the inferior vena cava. The right anterior cardinal and common cardinal veins form the superior vena cava. The left common cardinal vein forms the oblique vein of the heart.

27. VENA CAVAE AND CORONARY SINUS FORMATION (DORSAL ASPECT)

STAGE 12

STAGE 12 - 14

bulbus cordis (PR)

ventricle

atrium

sinus venosus (dB)

right common cardinal vein (dR)

umbilical vein (Y)

vitelline vein (lG)

left common cardinal vein (o)

STAGE 14

left common cardinal vein (o) (future oblique vein)

right common cardinal vein (dR)

sinus venosus (dB)

inferior vena cava (lG)

developing pulmonary veins (lB)

right vitelline vein (lG) (inferior vena cava)

STAGE 22

WEEK 11

superior vena cava (dR)

oblique vein of left atrium (o)

inferior vena cava (lG)

coronary sinus (o)

middle cardiac vein (o)

sinus venarum (dB)

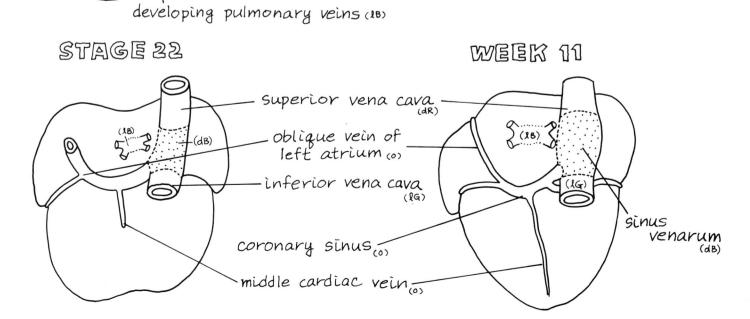

81

28. Ventricular Wall Formation

The early ventricular wall is composed of three layers; an outer myoepicardial mantle, a middle layer of cardiac jelly, and an inner layer of endothelial tissue. Ingrowths from the outer layer spread into the cardiac jelly. The endothelial tissue grows out and clothes the myoepicardial ingrowths with epithelium. The cardiac jelly disappears and the epithelial covered myoepicardial ingrowths form the trabeculae carneae, papillary muscles and chordae tendineae.

28. VENTRICULAR WALL FORMATION
STAGE 12

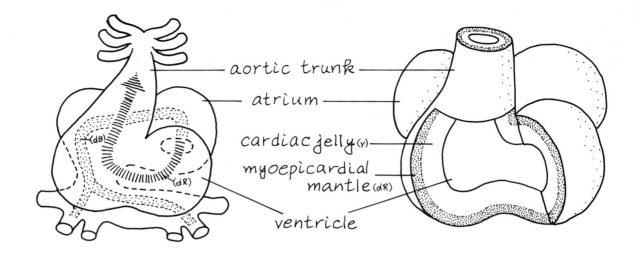

aortic trunk

atrium

cardiac jelly (Y)

myoepicardial mantle (dR)

ventricle

STAGE 12-13 STAGE 13-14

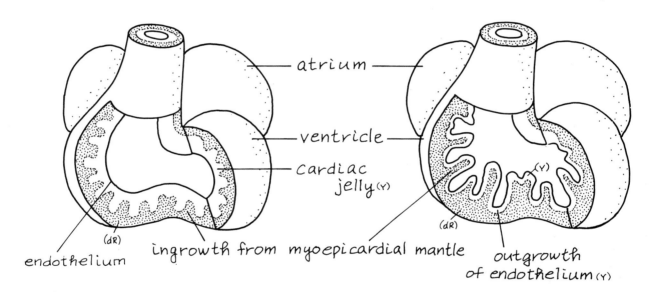

atrium

ventricle

cardiac jelly (Y)

endothelium

ingrowth from myoepicardial mantle

outgrowth of endothelium (Y)

29. Valve Formation

All of the valves of the heart form similarly. Subendocardial tissue swellings form at the sites of the future valves. These swellings subsequently hollow out to form cusps.

The valves of the aorta and truncus arteriosus form as the spiral septum separates the two vessels. Originally four endocardial cushions arise; but two of the four cushions are pinched and divided in half as the vessels form resulting in two sets of tricuspid valves.

29 . VALVE FORMATION
SEMILUNAR VALVES

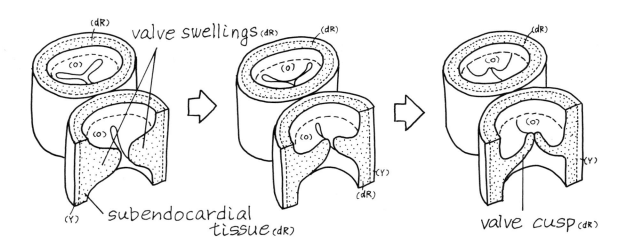

valve swellings (dR)

(dR)　(dR)　(dR)

subendocardial tissue (dR)

valve cusp (dR)

AORTA AND TRUNCUS ARTERIOSUS

STAGE 15~16

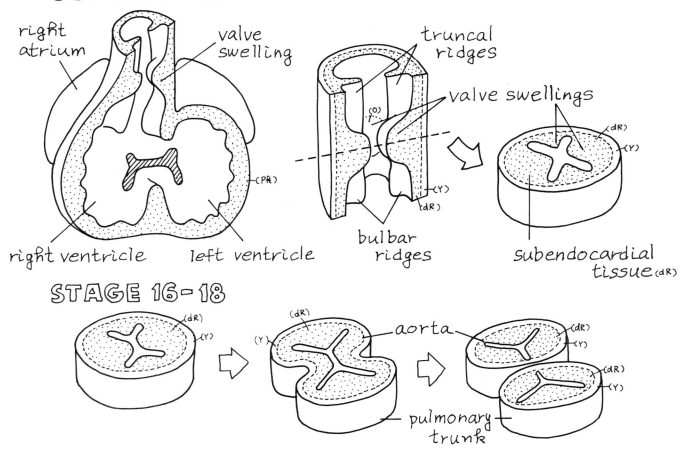

right atrium

valve swelling

truncal ridges

valve swellings

right ventricle　left ventricle

bulbar ridges

subendocardial tissue (dR)

STAGE 16~18

aorta

pulmonary trunk

30. Fetal Blood Flow Through the Heart

Before Birth

There are three shunts in the fetal cardiovascular system which cause blood to bypass the liver and lungs.

Liver Bypass

Blood returning from the placenta in the umbilical vein is well oxygenated. As it enters the fetus, approximately half is directed through the portal sinus to the portal vein and through the hepatic sinusoids. This blood then drains into the inferior vena cava. The other half of the umbilical vein blood bypasses the liver by entering the ductus venosus and passing into the inferior vena cava.

Lung Bypass

In the inferior vena cava, deoxygenated blood from the lower limbs, abdomen, and pelvis mixes with oxygenated umbilical vein blood and blood from the hepatic sinusoids. Upon entering the right atrium of the heart, most is directed through the foramen ovale by the inferior border of the septum secundum (crista dividens).

After the blood passes through the foramen ovale and enters into the left atrium, it mixes with a small amount of deoxygenated blood returning from the uninflated lungs. The blood then passes into the left ventricle and into the ascending aorta to supply the heart, head and neck, and upper limbs.

Other Lung Bypass

A small amount of oxygenated blood in the right atrium mixes with deoxygenated blood from the superior vena cava and coronary sinus. It passes to the right ventricle and into the pulmonary trunk. Because of high pulmonary resistance, most of this blood bypasses the lungs and passes through the ductus arteriosus into the aorta. Approximately half of this blood supplies the abdomen, pelvis, and lower limbs and half returns via the two umbilical arteries to the placenta and is re-oxygenated.

30. FETAL BLOOD FLOW THROUGH THE HEART

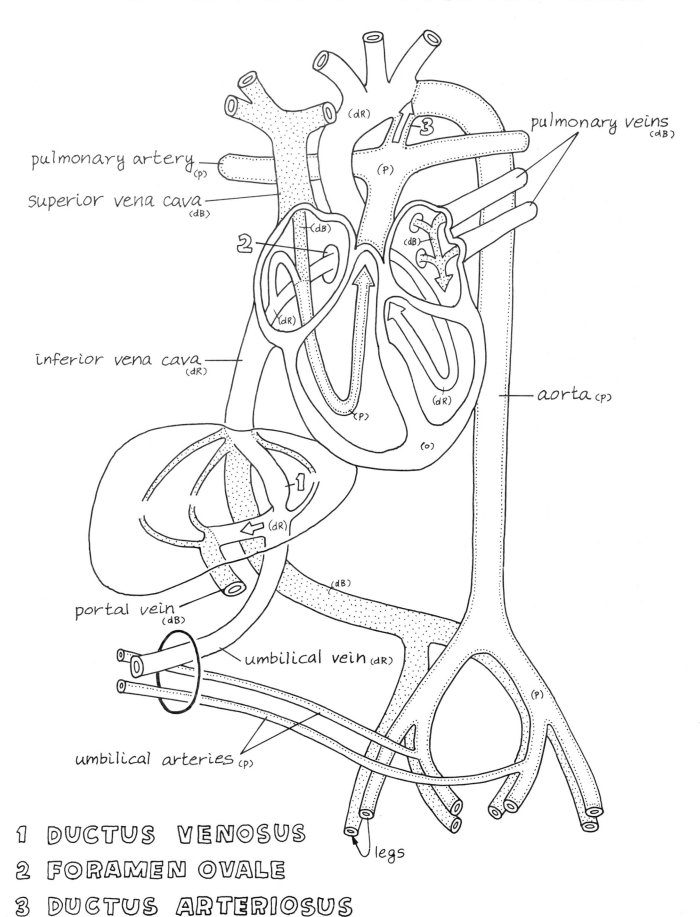

(dR)

pulmonary veins (dB)

pulmonary artery (p)

superior vena cava (dB)

(dB)

(P)

(dB)

(dB)

2

inferior vena cava (dR)

(dR)

(dR)

(P)

aorta (p)

(o)

1

(dR)

(dB)

portal vein (dB)

umbilical vein (dR)

(P)

umbilical arteries (p)

legs

1 DUCTUS VENOSUS
2 FORAMEN OVALE
3 DUCTUS ARTERIOSUS

31. Changes at Birth

At birth, the lungs expand and pulmonary resistance is reduced. This means that a greatly increased blood flow passes through the pulmonary arteries to the lungs. The ductus arteriosus then closes and will eventually degenerate to form the fibrous ligamentum arteriosum of the adult. The ductus arteriosus can remain patent as a developmental anomaly.

Blood returning through the pulmonary veins into the left atrium causes an increase in pressure in the left atrium. The septum primum is pressed against the septum secundum and the foramen ovale is functionally closed. In the adult, the site of the former septum primum is the floor of the fossa ovalis and the site of the former inferior edge of the septum secundum is located at the limbus fossae ovalis (anulus ovalis).

During postnatal development, most of the umbilical vessels within the infant become ligamentous; the umbilical vein forming the ligamentum teres, and the umbilical arteries distally forming the medial umbilical ligaments. Proximally the arteries persist as the superior vesical arteries. In the liver, the site of the ductus venosus can be recognised as the ligamentum venosum.

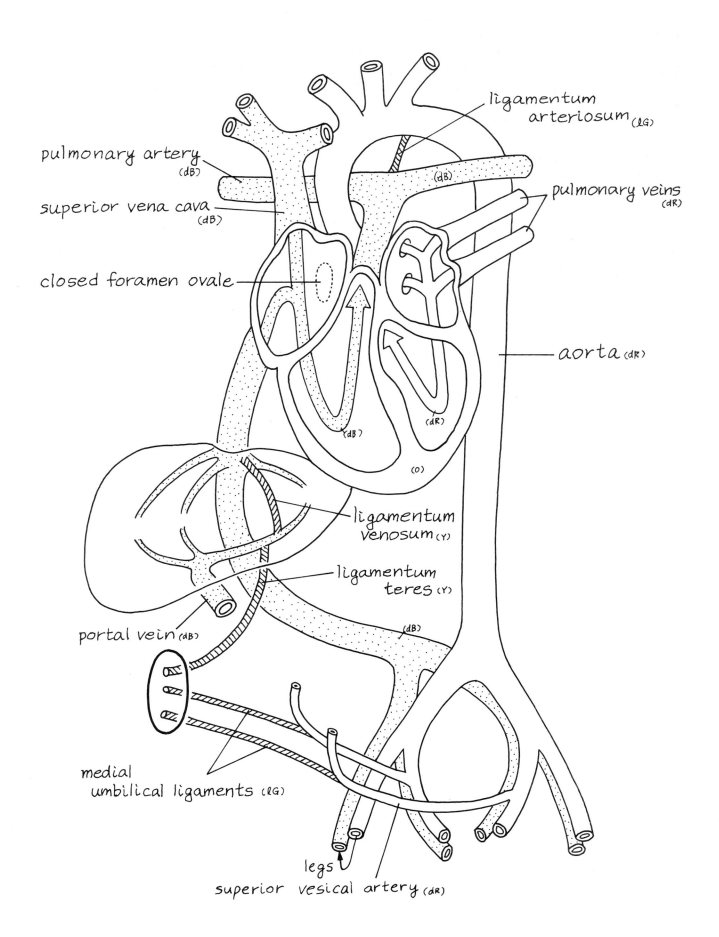

ligamentum arteriosum (LG)

pulmonary artery (dB)

superior vena cava (dB)

closed foramen ovale

(dB)

ligamentum venosum (Y)

ligamentum teres (Y)

portal vein (dB)

medial umbilical ligaments (LG)

ligamentum arteriosum (LG)

pulmonary veins (dR)

aorta (dR)

(dR)

(O)

(dB)

legs

superior vesical artery (dR)

32. Congenital Malformations of the Heart

Atrial Septal Defect

This anomaly is due to the persistence of the foramen ovale. The opening remains between the right and left atria due either to underdevelopment of the septum secundum, to excessive absorption of septum primum or to a combination of these two processes.

Ventricular Septal Defect

Interventricular septal defects are the most common congenital heart defect. They are usually found in the membranous part of the interventricular septum. This defect occurs when subendocardial tissue from the right side of the fused endocardial cushions fails to grow and fuse with the aorticopulmonary septum and the muscular part of the interventricular septum.

Tetralogy of Fallot

The anomalous formation of the aorticopulmonary septum can result in the tetralogy of Fallot which includes pulmonary valve stenosis, an overriding aorta, a ventricular septal defect and hypertrophy of the right ventricle. Other abnormalities may include a persistent truncus arteriosus or transposition of the great vessels.

32. CONGENITAL HEART MALFORMATION

NORMAL

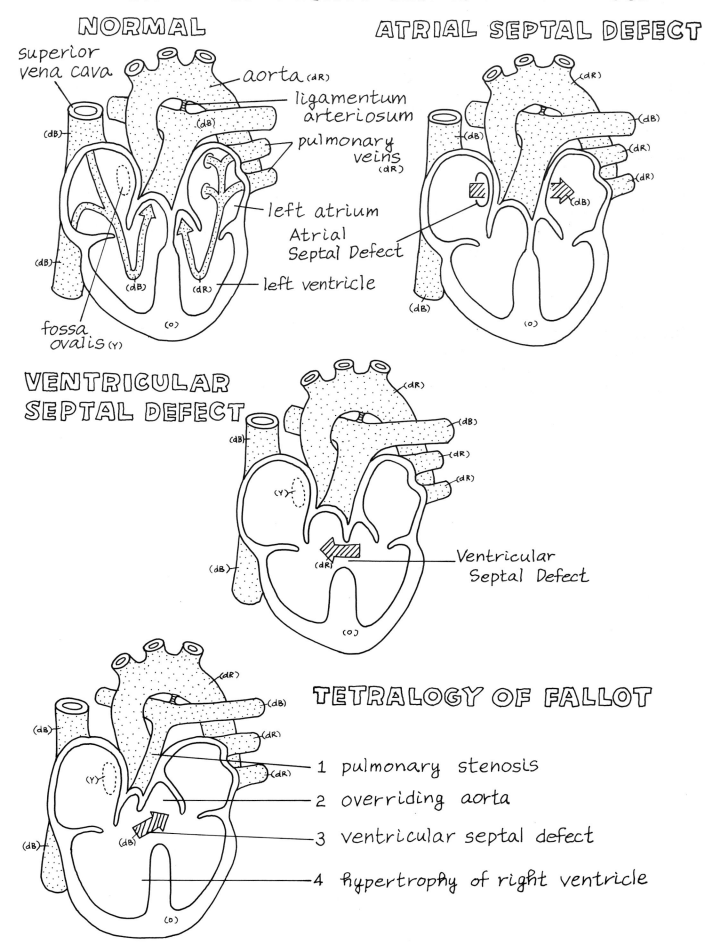

superior vena cava

aorta (dR)

ligamentum arteriosum

pulmonary veins (dR)

(dB)

(dB)

(dB)

left atrium

Atrial Septal Defect

left ventricle

fossa ovalis (Y)

(dB)

(dR)

(O)

ATRIAL SEPTAL DEFECT

(dR)

(dB)

(dR)

(dR)

(dB)

(dB)

(O)

VENTRICULAR SEPTAL DEFECT

(dR)

(dB)

(dB)

(dR)

(dR)

(Y)

(dB)

(dR)

Ventricular Septal Defect

(O)

TETRALOGY OF FALLOT

(dR)

(dB)

(dB)

(dR)

(dR)

(Y)

(dB)

(dB)

1 pulmonary stenosis

2 overriding aorta

3 ventricular septal defect

4 hypertrophy of right ventricle

(O)

NERVOUS SYSTEM

The first major system to develop is the nervous system and its primordia which appear in the early embryo in Week 3, Day 18. First the neural plate forms, followed by the neural folds and neural tube (neurulation). They will later give rise to the brain and spinal cord (central nervous system).

33. Early Neurulation

During early neurulation, the notochord and adjacent paraxial mesoderm cause or induce the overlying ectoderm to thicken and form neuroectoderm. This thickened neuroectoderm (neural plate) will form the brain and spinal cord.

The neural plate then bends in the midline to form a 'U' shape with the neural groove lying adjacent to the notochord and the neural folds forming the arms of the 'U'. By the beginning of Week 4, the neural folds approach one another in the medial plane and fuse first in the region between the brain and cervical spinal cord (at the level of the fourth to sixth somites). Fusion then proceeds both cephalically and caudally.

Fusion of the neural folds continues until only the two ends of the neural tube remain open: the rostral (anterior) neuropore and the caudal (posterior) neuropore. The rostral neuropore closes about Days 25–26 and the caudal one about Day 27.

Neural Crest

As the neural tube fuses, a region of the neuroectoderm located between the future neural tube and the surface ectoderm separates to form the neural crest. The neural crest will form the majority of the peripheral nervous system. This includes the autonomic nervous system, some of the cranial ganglia and spinal ganglia and the peripheral and cranial nerves. In addition, the neural crest cells give rise to parafollicular cells, the medulla (chromaffin cells) of the adrenal cortex, Schwann cells, the meninges, pigment cells, odontoblasts and numerous muscular and skeletal elements of the head.

NERVOUS SYSTEM

33. EARLY NEURULATION

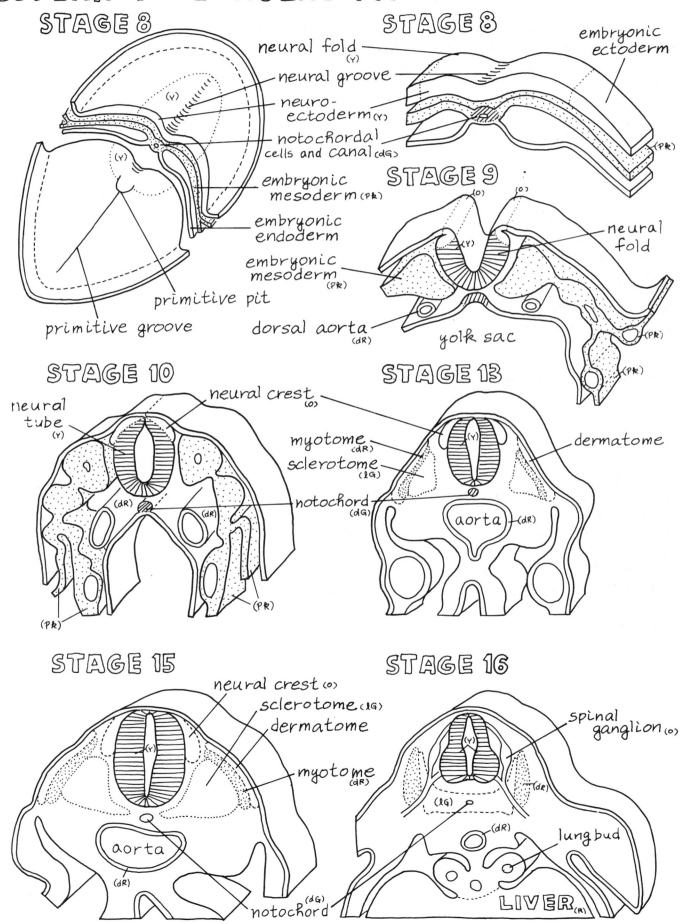

STAGE 8

primitive groove

primitive pit

STAGE 8

neural fold (Y)

neural groove

neuro-ectoderm (Y)

notochordal cells and canal (dG)

embryonic mesoderm (PR)

embryonic endoderm

embryonic ectoderm

(PR)

STAGE 9

embryonic mesoderm (PR)

dorsal aorta (dR)

neural fold

(O) (O)

(Y)

yolk sac

(PR)

(PR)

STAGE 10

neural tube (Y)

neural crest (O)

(dR) (dR)

(PR) (PR)

STAGE 13

myotome (dR)

sclerotome (lG)

notochord (dG)

dermatome

(Y)

aorta (dR)

STAGE 15

neural crest (O)

sclerotome (lG)

dermatome

myotome (dR)

(Y)

aorta (dR)

notochord (dG)

STAGE 16

spinal ganglion (O)

(Y)

(lG)

(dR)

lung bud

LIVER (R)

34. Early Histology of Spinal Cord

The spinal cord develops from the neural tube caudal to the fourth somite. This simple tube consists of a lumen called the central canal, with the walls initially composed of neuroepithelial cells. By Weeks 9–10 the walls have thickened and reduced the central canal to a small lumen.

The neural tube is initially composed of a pseudostratified columnar neuroepithelium. This neuroepithelium will form the ventricular (ependymal) zone which will give rise to all the spinal cord neurons and macroglia. Cells undergoing mitosis are evident along the internal limiting membrane of the luminal margin.

A second zone soon becomes evident along the border of the external limiting membrane. This marginal zone is composed of the outer parts of the neuroepithelial cells. This zone will eventually form the white matter of the spinal cord.

A third zone develops as the ventricular neuroepithelial cells continue to divide and produce neuroblasts or primitive neurons. These cells form an intermediate zone between the ventricular and marginal zones. Towards the end of neuroblast formation, the ventricular zone also produces glioblasts or primitive macroglial cells. These cells are the supporting cells of the spinal cord and will eventually form astrocytes or oligodendrocytes. Microglial cells are derivatives of the mesenchyme and migrate into the central nervous system in the late fetal period.

When the production of neuroblasts and glioblasts ceases, the neuroepithelial cells differentiate to form the ependymal lining of the central canal.

34. EARLY HISTOLOGY OF SPINAL CORD
STAGE 10

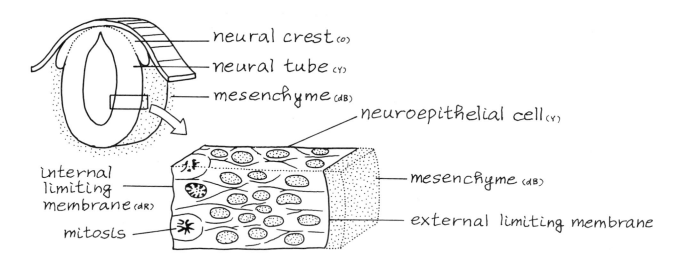

neural crest (O)

neural tube (Y)

mesenchyme (dB)

neuroepithelial cell (Y)

internal limiting membrane (dR)

mesenchyme (dB)

external limiting membrane

mitosis

STAGE 16

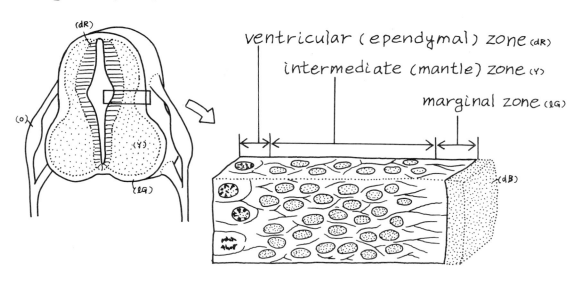

(dR)

(O)

(Y)

(lG)

ventricular (ependymal) zone (dR)

intermediate (mantle) zone (Y)

marginal zone (lG)

(dB)

DEVELOPMENT OF THE NEUROBLAST

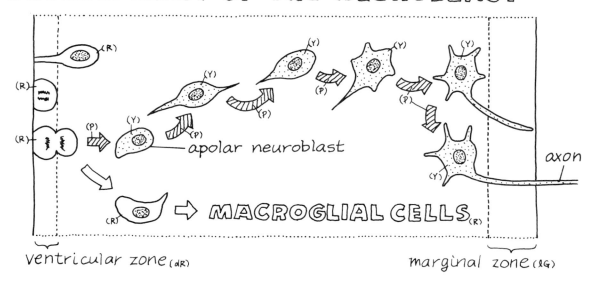

(R)

(R)

(R)

(P)

(Y)

(Y)

(Y)

(Y)

(Y)

(P)

(P)

(P)

(P)

(Y)

apolar neuroblast

(Y)

axon

(R)

MACROGLIAL CELLS (R)

ventricular zone (dR)

marginal zone (lG)

35. Spinal Cord: Alar and Basal Plates; and Spinal Nerves

As the neuroepithelial cells of the spinal cord proliferate, the walls of the cord become thickened, whilst the roof and floor plates remain thin. The central canal then becomes reduced in size, as the walls thicken, and a groove, the sulcus limitans, separates the dorsal wall or alar plate (alar lamina) from the ventral wall or basal plate (basal lamina).

35. SPINAL CORD AND SPINAL NERVES

STAGE 13

STAGE 13

neural crest (O)
(developing
spinal nerve)

dermatome

vitelline
vessel

neural tube (Y)

myotome (Pk)

sclerotome (dG)

aorta (dR)

notochord

STAGE 16

STAGE 16

spinal
ganglion
and
spinal nerve
(O)

spinal cord (Y)

(Pk)

(dG)

aorta (dR)

lung bud

(B)

LIVER

(R)

STAGE 19

STAGE 19

neural arch (dG)

scapula (dG)

body of
vertebra

oesophagus

trachea (B)

(Y)

(O)

(dG)

aortic arch (dR)

The alar plate is afferent in function and its cell bodies form columns of dorsal grey matter which run longitudinally in the cord. The dorsal grey columns are composed of groups of afferent nuclei which are composed of groups of neurons. In transverse sections of the cord, this area is called the dorsal grey horn

The basal plate is efferent in function and its cell bodies form ventral and lateral grey columns. Axons from the ventral grey columns grow out to form the ventral roots of the spinal nerves. In a transverse section of the cord, the ventral and lateral columns are called the ventral and lateral grey horns. The lateral horn, containing the cells of origin of the sympathetic system, is present in sections of vertebral levels T1 or T2 to L2. The dorsal root (spinal) ganglia are neural crest derivatives. The axons of cells in these ganglia are bipolar, but soon change to form a 'T' shape. The peripheral processes pass in the spinal nerve, while the central ones enter the spinal cord as the dorsal root of the spinal nerve.

STAGE 13

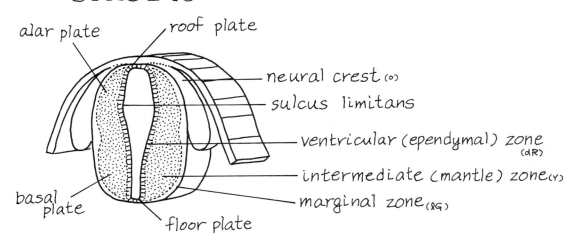

alar plate

roof plate

neural crest (o)

sulcus limitans

ventricular (ependymal) zone (dR)

intermediate (mantle) zone (Y)

basal plate

marginal zone (lG)

floor plate

STAGE 16

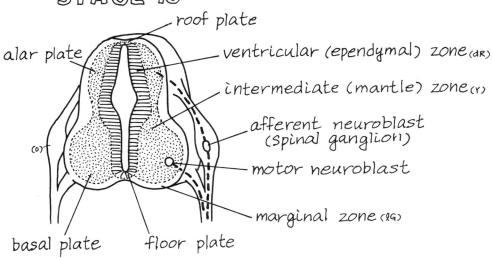

roof plate

alar plate

ventricular (ependymal) zone (dR)

intermediate (mantle) zone (Y)

afferent neuroblast (spinal ganglion)

motor neuroblast

(o)

marginal zone (lG)

basal plate   floor plate

STAGE 19

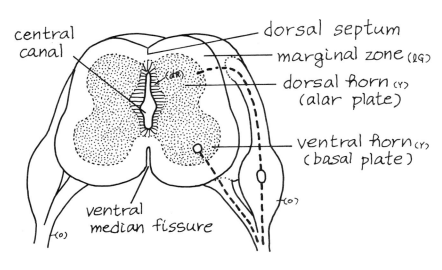

central canal

dorsal septum

marginal zone (lG)

dorsal horn (Y) (alar plate)

(dR)

ventral horn (Y) (basal plate)

ventral median fissure

(o)

(o)

Ascent of the Spinal Cord

Initially the spinal cord and the three layers of the meninges occupy the entire length of the vertebral canal. The spinal nerves come directly off the spinal cord and emerge through the vertebral foramina of the vertebrae immediately adjacent to them.

As the surrounding vertebral column and the dura mater grow more rapidly than the spinal cord, the spinal cord appears to 'ascend' in the vertebral canal. At birth, the spinal cord terminates at approximately the level of L2–L3 vertebrae. In the adult, the spinal cord ends at approximately L1–L2. The end of the cord becomes the adult conus medullaris.

As a result of this 'ascent', the spinal nerves emerge from the cord to run obliquely to their vertebral foramina. Those nerves in the lumbar and sacral regions come to form the cauda equina. The pia mater which is attached proximally to the conus medullaris, becomes drawn out into a long thread, the filum terminale. This marks the line of the regressing spinal cord. Distally, the filum is attached to the periosteum of the first coccygeal vertebra. The dura and arachnoid mater extend to S2 in the adult.

ASCENT OF THE SPINAL CORD
STAGE 23

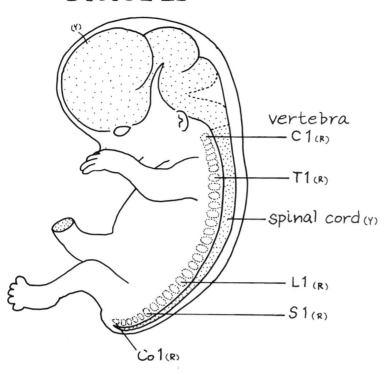

vertebra
C 1 (R)

T1 (R)

spinal cord (Y)

L1 (R)

S 1 (R)

Co 1 (R)

WEEK 8   WEEK 24   NEW BORN

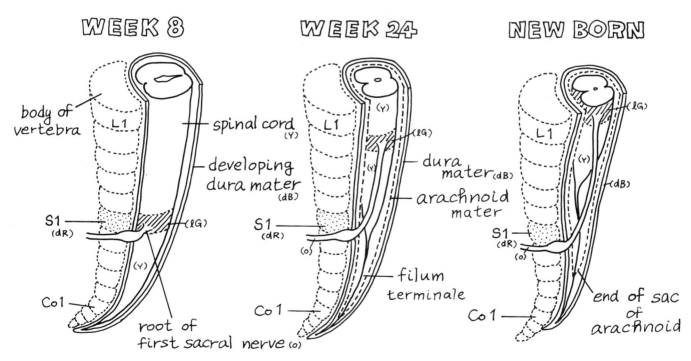

body of vertebra

L1

spinal cord (Y)

developing dura mater (dB)

S1 (dR)

(ℓG)

(Y)

Co1

root of first sacral nerve (o)

L1

(Y)

(ℓG)

dura mater (dB)

arachnoid mater

S1 (dR)

(o)

filum terminale

Co 1

(ℓG)

L1

(Y)

(dB)

S1 (dR)

(o)

Co 1

end of sac of arachnoid

36. Brain: Early Development

The neural tube fuses initially between somites 4 and 6 and the brain will form rostral to somite 4. Even before the neural tube fuses, the site of the future primary vesicles is identifiable as large, elevated cephalic neural folds. In Stage 11, the primary vesicles develop and become the prosencephalon (forebrain), the mesencephalon (midbrain) and the large rhombencephalon (hindbrain). The neural folds in the brain region have fused (except for the rostral neuropore) and the three main brain vesicles are present.

By Stage 13, two of the three primary vesicles have subdivided to form five major regions. The prosencephalon (forebrain) has divided into two areas: the telencephalon from which the cerebral vesicles will arise and the most caudal diencephalon. The mesencephalon (midbrain) region remains undivided; while the rhombencephalon has divided into two parts: the metencephalon and myelencephalon. The pons and cerebellum will form in the metencephalon, while the myelencephalon which is continuous with the spinal cord will give rise to the medulla oblongata.

As the brain grows rapidly, it begins to fold upon itself and three major flexures are formed (see **38**. Ventricle Formation and Folding of the Brain).

36. BRAIN: EARLY DEVELOPMENT

STAGE 10

STAGE 11

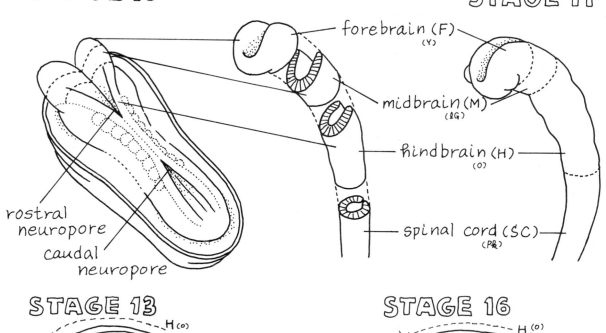

forebrain (F)
(Y)

midbrain (M)
(lG)

hindbrain (H)
(O)

spinal cord (SC)
(Pk)

rostral neuropore

caudal neuropore

STAGE 13

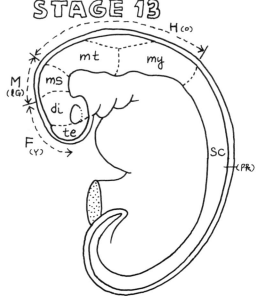

H (O)

mt

my

M (lG)

ms

di

te

F (Y)

SC
(Pk)

STAGE 16

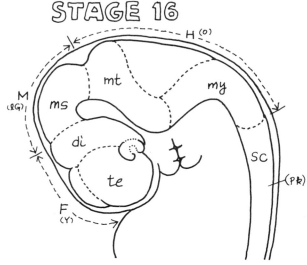

H (O)

mt

my

M (lG)

ms

di

te

SC
(Pk)

F (Y)

STAGE 19

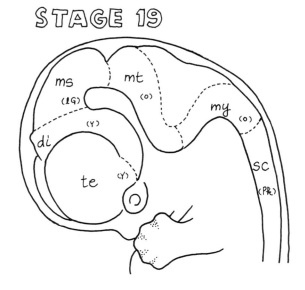

ms
(lG)

mt
(O)

my
(O)

di

(Y)

te
(Y)

SC
(Pk)

STAGE 23

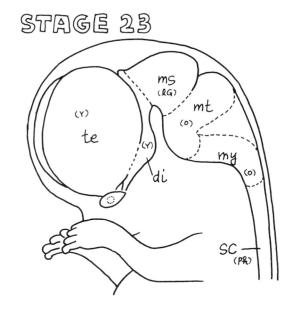

ms
(lG)

mt
(O)

te
(Y)

(Y)

di

my
(O)

SC
(Pk)

37. Growth of Cerebral Vesicles and Meninges

The two outgrowths of the telencephalon, the cerebral vesicles, grow rapidly and as the future cerebral hemispheres expand to successively cover the diencephalon, midbrain, and hindbrain. As the hemispheres' cortical surfaces grow more rapidly than the floor, the expanding hemispheres become 'C' shaped. The ventricles within the hemispheres also become 'C' shaped.

The caudal end of each hemisphere then turns ventrally and rostrally to form the temporal lobe. As the temporal lobe grows forward, it and the lips of the frontal and parietal lobes grow and bury a region of cortex called the insula. As the temporal lobe grows over the insula, it carries the temporal horn of the ventricle into its final position and the lateral sulcus is formed The occipital lobe develops when the posterior part of each hemisphere grows caudally.

The surface of the cerebral hemispheres is initially smooth, but by Week 18 the surface begins to acquire a characteristic pattern of grooves or furrows called sulci and a pattern of convolutions called gyri. The central sulcus delineates the motor area rostrally and the sensory area caudally.

37. BRAIN: GROWTH OF CEREBRAL VESICLES AND MENINGES

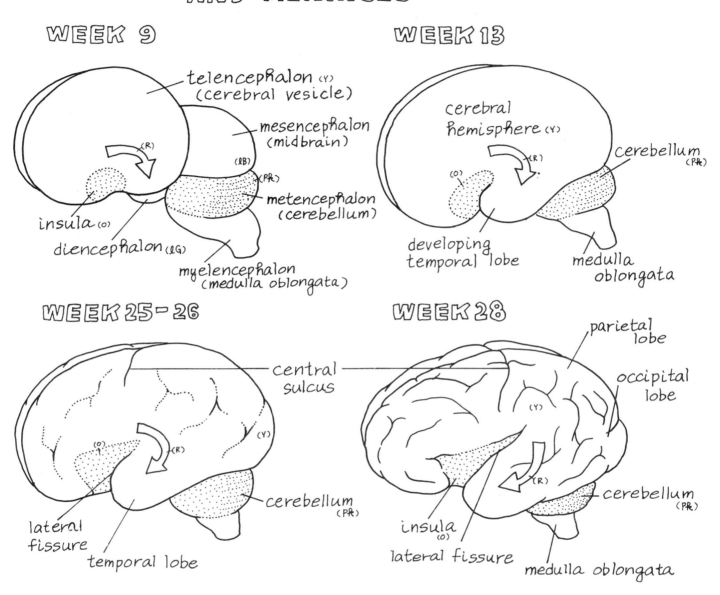

WEEK 9

telencephalon (Y)
(cerebral vesicle)

mesencephalon
(midbrain)

(lB)

(PR)

metencephalon
(cerebellum)

(R)

insula (O)

diencephalon (lG)

myelencephalon
(medulla oblongata)

WEEK 13

cerebral hemisphere (Y)

cerebellum
(PR)

(O)

(R)

developing temporal lobe

medulla oblongata

WEEK 25-26

central sulcus

(O)

(R)

(Y)

cerebellum
(PR)

lateral fissure

temporal lobe

WEEK 28

parietal lobe

occipital lobe

(Y)

(R)

cerebellum
(PR)

insula
(O)

lateral fissure

medulla oblongata

The spinal meninges form from mesenchyme surrounding the spinal cord. The condensing mesenchyme or primitive meninx will form two main layers: an outer one which will form dura mater and an inner one which will form the leptomeninges, i.e. the pia and arachnoid maters. Neural crest cells contribute to the leptomeninges. The cranial dura mater forms in close association with the developing skull. Spaces filled with fluid appear in the leptomeninges; these then coalesce and form the subarachnoid space.

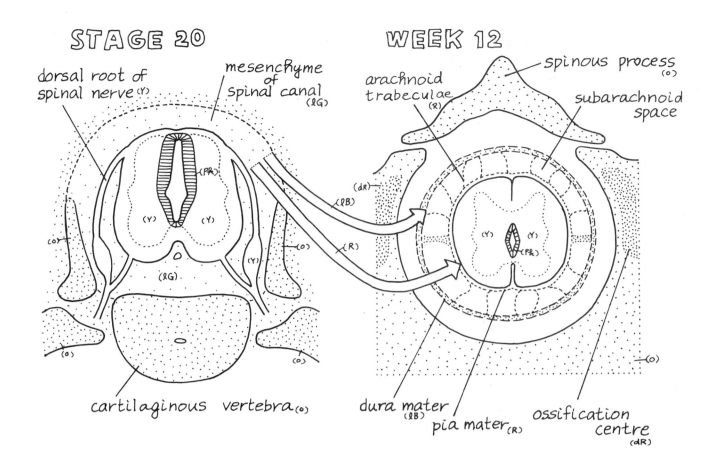

STAGE 20

dorsal root of
spinal nerve (Y)

mesenchyme
of
spinal canal
(ℓG)

(PR)

(Y)   (Y)

(O)

(O)

(ℓG)

(Y)

(O)

(O)

cartilaginous vertebra (O)

WEEK 12

arachnoid
trabeculae
(R)

spinous process
(O)

subarachnoid
space

(dR)

(ℓB)

(R)

(Y)   (Y)

(PR)

dura mater
(ℓB)

pia mater (R)

ossification
centre
(dR)

(O)

107

38. Ventricle Formation and Folding of the Brain

Initially the lumen of the neural tube is approximately the same size and shape throughout its length. However, the shape of the lumen changes with the formation of the flexures, and the cerebral hemispheres. Thickenings also develop in the walls of the neural tube. The resulting interconnected spaces in the brain are known as the ventricular system.

As already explained, the shapes of the ventricles are determined by the formation of the flexures. As the brain grows rapidly it bends (as does the lumen). The initial flexion in the region of the midbrain causes the midbrain flexure. A second flexion occurs between the brain and spinal cord, this is the cervical flexure which later disappears. Finally, the pontine flexure occurs in the hindbrain causing its walls to be splayed and its roof to thin greatly.

During development, the two lateral ventricles can be found in the two developing cerebral hemispheres. Each ventricle is continuous with the central third ventricle through a narrow interventricular foramen. The third ventricle is wide rostrally, and narrows caudally to form the cerebral aqueduct (of Sylvius). This is a direct result of the developing thalami bulging into this area. The cerebral aqueduct is continuous with the fourth ventricle. This ventricle is diamond-shaped as a direct result of the pontine flexure splaying the walls of the hindbrain. The fourth ventricle is continuous with the central lumen of the spinal cord.

Each ventricle develops a choroid plexus which produces cerebrospinal fluid (CSF). They all develop similarly; for example, the roof of the fourth ventricle is covered externally by mesenchyme which will form pia mater. As the vascularised pia mater then proliferates rapidly, it invaginates into the fourth ventricle and with the ependymal roof forms the tela choriodea and then choroid plexus. The CSF which is formed passes through the ventricular system and eventually escapes through three openings to bathe the outer surface of the brain and spinal cord. These three openings develop in the roof of the hindbrain, and are the median foramen (of Magendie) and the two lateral foramina (of Luschka). Programmed cell degeneration is responsible for the formation of the foramina, not the pressure of CSF rupturing the hindbrain roof.

The choroid plexus of the third ventricle also develops in the roof, while those of the lateral ventricles develop in the medial walls.

38. VENTRICLE FORMATION AND FOLDING OF THE BRAIN

STAGE 16

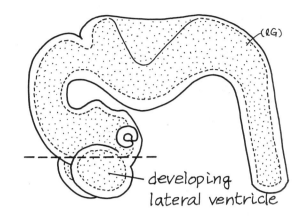

developing lateral ventricle

(lG)

STAGE 16

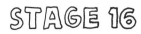

inter-ventricular foramen (R)

(dB)

(Y)

developing lateral ventricle

STAGE 23

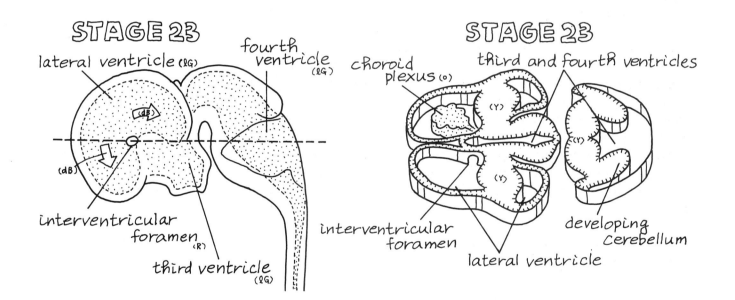

lateral ventricle (lG)

fourth ventricle (lG)

(dB)

(dB)

interventricular foramen (R)

third ventricle (lG)

STAGE 23

choroid plexus (o)

third and fourth ventricles

(Y)

(Y)

(Y)

interventricular foramen

lateral ventricle

developing Cerebellum

WEEK 12

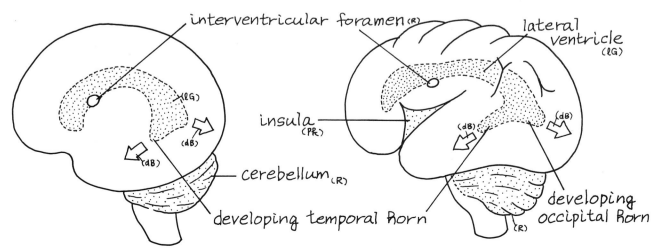

interventricular foramen (R)

(lG)

(dB)

(dB)

cerebellum (R)

developing temporal horn

WEEK 24

lateral ventricle (lG)

insula (PR)

(dB)

(dB)

developing occipital horn

(R)

39. Internal Capsule and Basal Ganglia

In the striatal part of the floor of each cerebral hemisphere, a swelling appears in Week 6 called the corpus striatum.

Fibres then develop which pass to and from the cerebral hemispheres. These fibres pass through the corpus striatum in a bundle called the internal capsule and they divide the corpus striatum into the medial caudate nucleus and lateral lentiform nucleus.

39. INTERNAL CAPSULE AND BASAL GANGLIA

STAGE 16

A

(dB) (O) (dG)

(R)

(Y)

(PR)

section
shown
in B

diencephalon

telencephalon

STAGE 16

B

diencephalon

third
ventricle

lateral
ventricle

striatal
part

(dR)

(Y)

nasal pit
(P)

HEART

STAGE 19

choroid
fissure

lateral
ventricle

choroid plexus

inter-
ventricular
foramen

striatal
ridge (dR)

third ventricle

(Y)

(B)

(B)

STAGE 20

lateral
ventricle

corpus
striatum
(dR)

thalamus (dR)

hypothalamus
(dR)

(Y)

(Y)

WEEK 10

lateral ventricle

choroid plexus (Y)

caudate nucleus (dR)

thalamus (dR)

lentiform nucleus (O)

internal capsule (lG)

hypothalamus (dR)

third
ventricle

The cerebral hemispheres then grow caudally, and the temporal lobe grows inferiorly and rostrally. This causes the internal capsule to become 'C' shaped and the caudate nucleus becomes elongated in the shape of the lateral ventricle.

ADULT

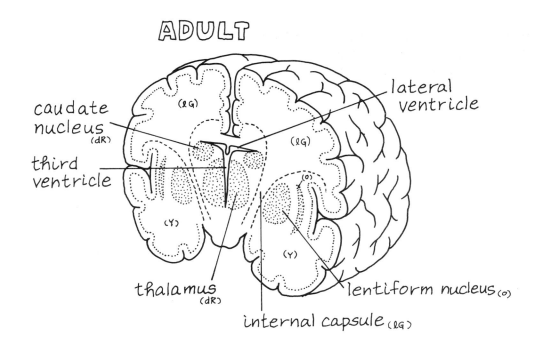

caudate
nucleus
(dR)

third
ventricle

lateral
ventricle

(lG)

(lG)

(o)

(Y)

(Y)

thalamus
(dR)

internal capsule (lG)

lentiform nucleus (o)

40. Histology of the Cerebral Cortex

Initially the neural tube of both the spinal cord and future brain is a pseudostratified neuroepithelium. The first layer formed is the ventricular zone with an internal limiting membrane adjacent to the lumen and an outer external limiting membrane. This layer in the cerebral cortex is penetrated by primitive corticopetal fibres which penetrate the entire layer. As these fibres pass horizontally, they establish an external layer of white matter termed the marginal zone or primordial plexiform layer. This layer appears by Stage 15 and is of short duration. While present, it is very active functionally and gives rise to the Cajal–Retzius cells and to the first synapses. The intermediate layer forms from immature neurons which have arisen from the ventricular zone and moved outwards.

The cortical plate arises at Stage 22 as migrating neuroblasts penetrate and accumulate within the primordial plexiform layer. This plate divides the plexiform layer into two layers whose numbering will follow that used to describe the layers of the adult brain: I (primitive superficial plexiform) and a deep layer VII (layer VI6) which ultimately will regress and disappear. Layer I will increase dramatically in vertical and horizontal thickness and will play an important role in the organisation of the adult cerebral cortex.

The cortical plate gives rise to the remaining layers in the order, VI, V, IV, III and II. This formation is an ascending 'inside-out' progression. Neuronal differentiation starts at layer VI and ascends through layers V, IV, III and II. The traditional view of the origin of the layers is the first layers to arise are V and VI, followed by IIIa and IV, and finally layers I and II. Recent evidence, however, supports the 'inside-out progression'.

The embryonic white matter consists of connections forming between cortical cells and other parts of the brain.

Cerebral Commissures

As the cerebral cortex develops, groups of fibres connect corresponding areas with one another. The first two to form are the anterior and hippocampal commissures which connect the phylogenetically older areas of the brain. The corpus callosum connects neocortical areas.

Neuroglia

Macroglia form from neuroepithelial cells of the ventricular zone. Microglia are small neuroglial cells present in the central nervous system from an early age (Weeks 5–8). There is much controversy surrounding their origin.

40. HISTOLOGY OF THE CEREBRAL CORTEX

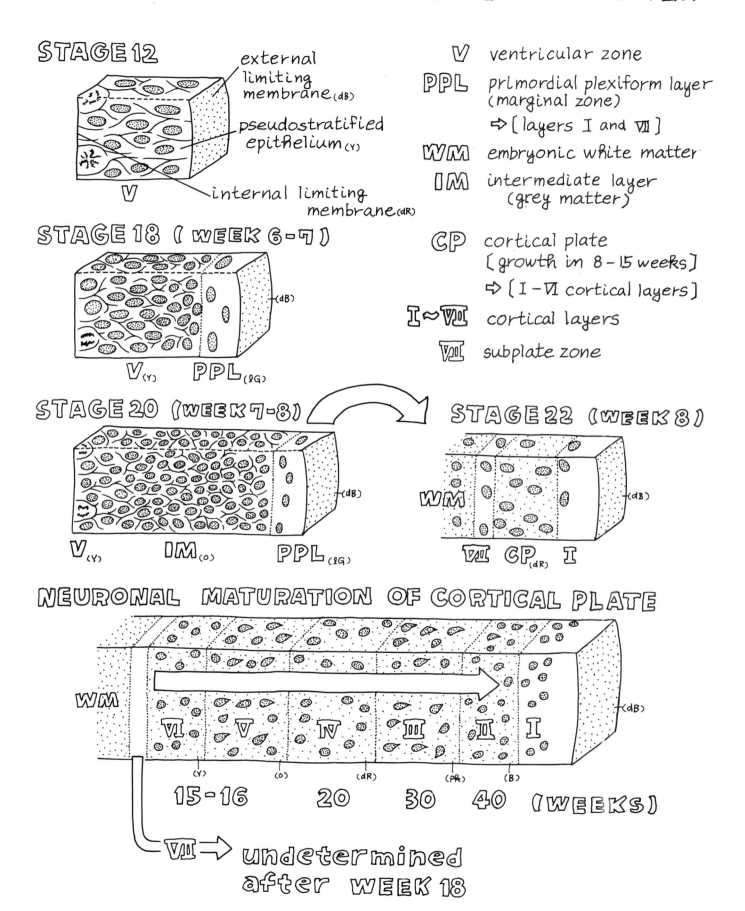

STAGE 12

external limiting membrane (dB)

pseudostratified epithelium (Y)

internal limiting membrane (dR)

V

STAGE 18 (WEEK 6-7)

(dB)

V (Y)   PPL (lG)

STAGE 20 (WEEK 7-8)

(dB)

V (Y)   IM (O)   PPL (lG)

STAGE 22 (WEEK 8)

WM

(dB)

VII CP (dR) I

V   ventricular zone
PPL   primordial plexiform layer (marginal zone)
      ⇨ [layers I and VII]
WM   embryonic white matter
IM   intermediate layer (grey matter)
CP   cortical plate [growth in 8-15 weeks]
      ⇨ [I - VI cortical layers]
I~VII cortical layers
VII   subplate zone

NEURONAL MATURATION OF CORTICAL PLATE

WM

(dB)

VI   V   IV   III   II   I

(Y)   (O)   (dR)   (PR)   (B)

15-16   20   30   40   (WEEKS)

VII ⇨ undetermined after WEEK 18

115

41. Diencephalon

The walls of the diencephalon thicken as three large swellings develop in each lateral wall. These three swellings are in order from superior to inferior, the epithalamus, thalamus and hypothalamus. All of these swellings bulge into the third ventricle and, in 70% of people, the two thalami meet and fuse in the midline to form the interthalamic adhesion.

At first, the epithalami are relatively large but decrease in size later. The mamillary bodies and several nuclei concerned with homeostasis and endocrine functions develop in the hypothalami. The pineal body forms in the roof of the caudal part of the diencephalon. The hypophysis or pituitary gland is also a derivative of the diencephalon (and stomodeal ectoderm) and is considered in **45**. Hypophysis Cerebri (Pituitary Gland).

41. DIENCEPHALON
STAGE 19

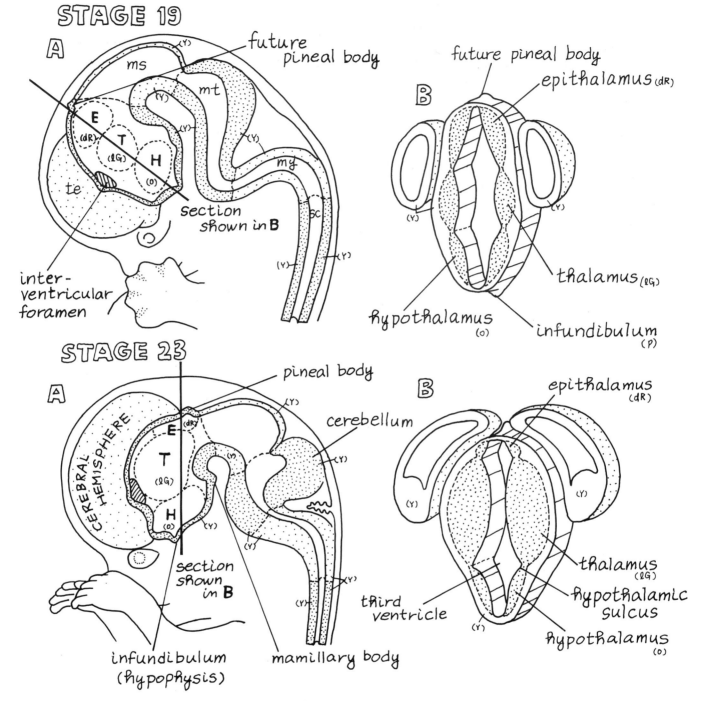

A
- ms
- mt
- future pineal body
- E (dR)
- T (ℓG)
- H
- te
- (o)
- section shown in B
- my
- sc
- inter-ventricular foramen

B
- future pineal body
- epithalamus (dR)
- thalamus (ℓG)
- hypothalamus (o)
- infundibulum (P)

STAGE 23

A
- CEREBRAL HEMISPHERE
- pineal body
- E (dR)
- T (ℓG)
- H (o)
- cerebellum
- section shown in B
- infundibulum (hypophysis)
- mamillary body

B
- epithalamus (dR)
- thalamus (ℓG)
- hypothalamic sulcus
- hypothalamus (o)
- third ventricle

E : epithalamus
T : thalamus
H : hypothalamus

te : telencephalon
ms : mesencephalon
mt : metencephalon
my : myelencephalon
sc : spinal cord

42. Midbrain

Several structures form in the walls of the mesencephalon (midbrain) causing them to thicken. As a result, the neural lumen narrows and forms the cerebral aqueduct.

Neuroblasts from the alar plate migrate into the tectum (roof) and form the paired superior colliculi (concerned with vision) and the paired inferior colliculi (concerned with auditory reflexes).

The tegmentum (floor) is thickened by the formation of the paired red nuclei, the reticular nuclei, the nuclei of the third and fourth cranial nerves, the substantia nigra, and the cerebral peduncles. The origins of the cells of the red nuclei, reticular nuclei and substantia nigra are in dispute. Some believe them to be of basal plate origin and others that they migrated from the alar plate. The cerebral peduncles form as fibres grow from the cerebrum and pass through the midbrain to the brain stem and spinal cord. These fibres form the corticobulbar, corticospinal and corticopontine tracts.

42. MIDBRAIN
STAGE 16

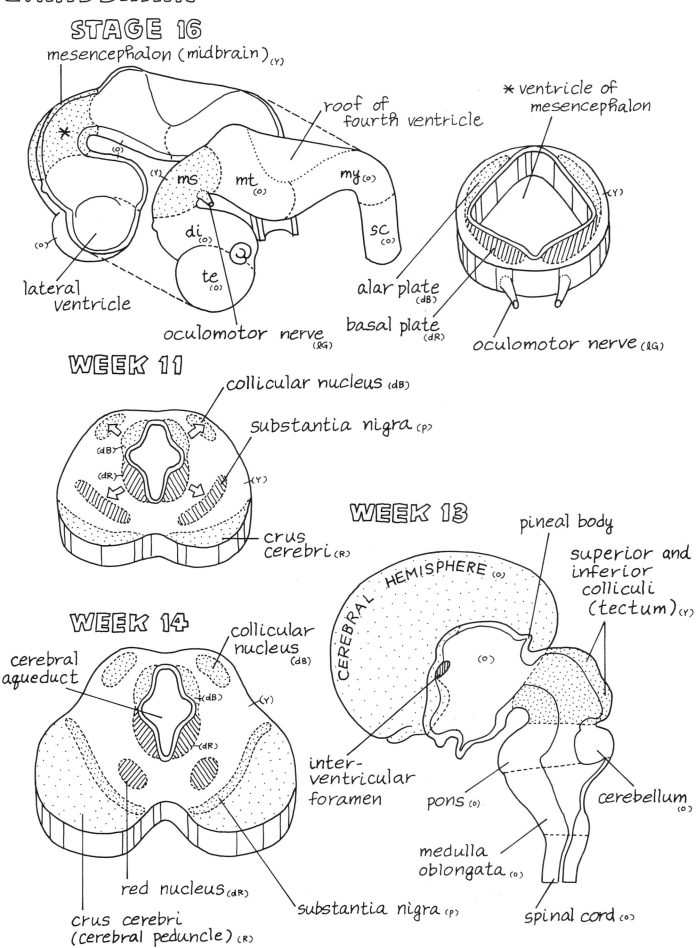

mesencephalon (midbrain) (Y)

roof of
fourth ventricle

* ventricle of
mesencephalon

ms

mt (O)

my (O)

SC (O)

(Y)

di (O)

te (O)

(O)

lateral
ventricle

oculomotor nerve (ℓG)

alar plate (dB)

basal plate (dR)

oculomotor nerve (ℓG)

WEEK 11

collicular nucleus (dB)

substantia nigra (P)

(dB)

(dR)

(Y)

crus
cerebri (R)

WEEK 13

pineal body

superior and
inferior
colliculi
(tectum) (Y)

CEREBRAL HEMISPHERE (O)

(O)

WEEK 14

collicular
nucleus (dB)

cerebral
aqueduct

(dB)

(Y)

(dR)

inter-
ventricular
foramen

pons (O)

cerebellum (O)

red nucleus (dR)

medulla
oblongata (O)

crus cerebri
(cerebral peduncle) (R)

substantia nigra (P)

spinal cord (O)

43. Pons and Medulla Oblongata

The pons and cerebellum are derivatives of the metencephalon (see **44**. Cerebellum). The myelencephalon gives rise to the medulla oblongata. With the appearance of the pontine flexure, the caudal part of the metencephalon and the rostral part of the myelencephalon become splayed. The hindbrain roof becomes very thin over the lumen of the future fourth ventricle. This diamond-shaped ventricle is continuous caudally with the central canal of the caudal myelencephalon and spinal cord. As the walls splay, the alar plates of the pons and medulla oblongata come to lie lateral to the basal plates. This is why the motor nuclei come to lie medial to the sensory nuclei. From lateral to medial, the alar plate cell columns are: special somatic afferent, general somatic afferent, special visceral afferent, general visceral afferent. The motor plate cell columns are: general visceral efferent, special visceral efferent, general somatic efferent. The pontine and olivary nuclei form when neuroblasts from the alar plate migrate ventrally.

A choroid plexus develops in the roof of the fourth ventricle.

Further caudally, where the medulla oblongata no longer has a thin roof, the fourth ventricle is continuous with the central canal. In the dorsal part of the medulla at this level are two areas of grey matter, the gracile nuclei medially and the cuneate nuclei laterally. These nuclei are formed from neuroblasts migrating from the alar plates. Corticospinal fibres form the pyramid in the ventral part of the medulla at this level.

43. PONS AND MEDULLA OBLONGATA

STAGE 15

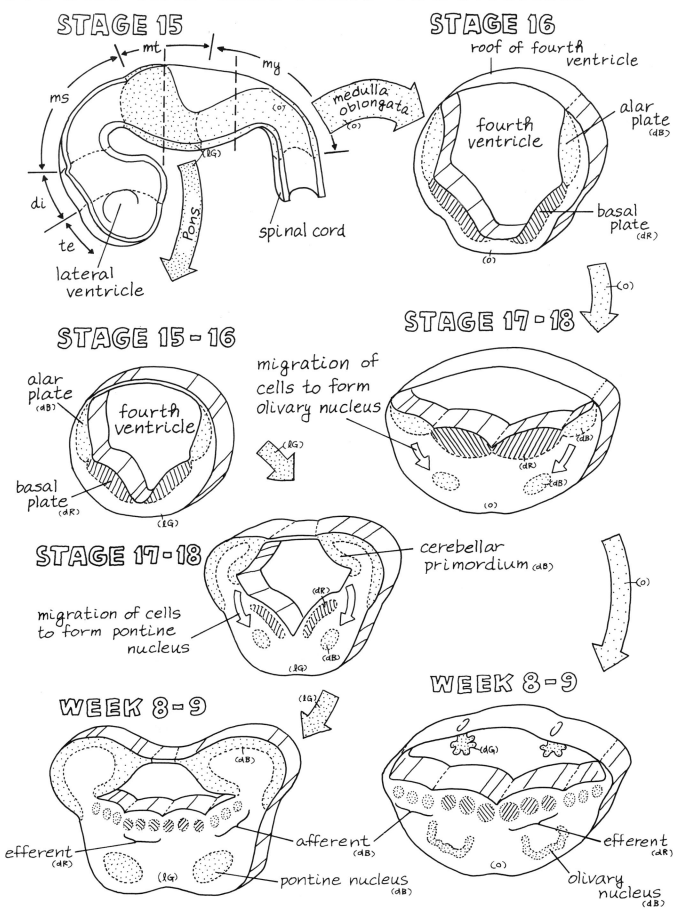

mt

my

ms

(o)

di

te

(ℓG)

lateral
ventricle

medulla
oblongata
(o)

Pons

spinal cord

STAGE 16

roof of fourth
ventricle

fourth
ventricle

alar
plate
(dB)

basal
plate
(dR)

(o)

(o)

STAGE 15-16

alar
plate
(dB)

fourth
ventricle

basal
plate
(dR)

(ℓG)

(ℓG)

STAGE 17-18

migration of
cells to form
olivary nucleus

(ℓG)

(dB)

(dR)

(dB)

(o)

STAGE 17-18

migration of cells
to form pontine
nucleus

cerebellar
primordium (dB)

(dR)

(dB)

(ℓG)

(o)

WEEK 8-9

(ℓG)

(dB)

efferent
(dR)

(ℓG)

afferent
(dB)

pontine nucleus
(dB)

WEEK 8-9

(dG)

afferent
(dB)

(o)

efferent
(dR)

olivary
nucleus
(dB)

In the adult pons and medulla oblongata the afferent columns lie lateral to the efferent columns.

The pyramids of the medulla oblongata are composed of corticospinal fibres descending from the cerebral cortex.

PONS (ADULT)

MEDULLA (ADULT)

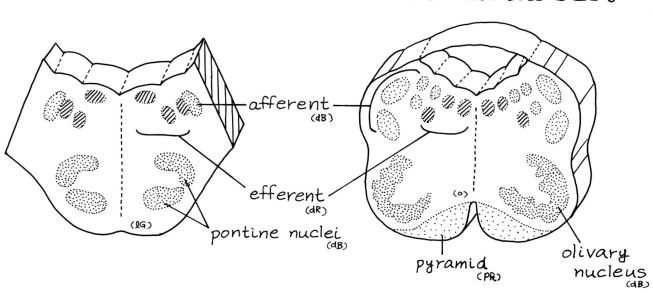

afferent
(dB)

efferent
(dR)

pontine nuclei
(dB)

(lG)

(o)

pyramid
(PR)

olivary
nucleus
(dB)

44. Cerebellum

The cerebellum forms from two thickenings in the roof of the metencephalon (the dorsal parts of the alar plates). The thickenings project both into the fourth ventricle, as well as on the surface of the metencephalon. The two cerebellar projections meet and fuse in the midline forming a dumb-bell shape, which then enlarges and overgrows the rostral half of the fourth ventricle, the pons and medulla oblongata.

The lateral parts of the cerebellum enlarge to form lobes and in the fourth month fissures develop in these lobes.

Neuroblasts from the alar plates form the neurons of the cerebellar cortex and also give rise to the central nuclei (e.g. dentate nucleus), and the pontine, vestibular and cochlear nuclei, and the sensory nuclei of the trigeminal nerve.

44. CEREBELLUM

STAGE 16

cerebellar primordium (O)

(PR)

(PR)

roof of 4th ventricle

STAGE 17 - 18

(dB)

(PR)

intra-ventricular portion (O)

4th ventricle

extra-ventricular portion (O)

WEEK 12

(PR)
(Y)
(O)

postero-lateral fissure

choroid fissure

median aperture

(PR)

primary fissure

nodulus (lG)

flocculus (lG)

4th ventricle

choroid plexus (dG)

(PR)

(Y)
(O)

primary fissure

(lG)

(PR)

primordium of dentate nucleus (dR)

WEEK 14 - 16

cerebellar cortex

primary fissure

(PR)

(Y)
(O)

4th ventricle

(PR)

dentate nucleus (dR)

nodulus (lG)

(dG)

WEEK 16

pyramid

lingula (Y)

(PR)
(Y)
(O)

primary fissure

secondary fissure

flocculus (lG)

nodulus (lG)

(PR)

uvula (O)

WEEK 18 - 19

anterior lobe (Y)

posterior lobe (O)

flocculo-nodular lobe (lG)

pons (PR)

(PR)

olive (R)

45. Hypophysis Cerebri (Pituitary Gland)

The parts of the hypophysis cerebri (pituitary gland) have separate derivations, partly as a diverticulum from the roof of the primitive mouth cavity (Rathke's pouch) and partly as a diverticulum from the diencephalon (infundibulum).

In the middle of Week 4, the two diverticulae grow towards each other and in Week 7 they join to form the hypophysis.

Those parts of the pituitary gland formed from Rathke's pouch are the glandular portion: pars anterior, pars intermedia, pars distalis and pars tuberalis and are collectively called the adenohypophysis. The part formed from the infundibulum is the nervous portion or neurohypophysis. This includes the median eminence, infundibular stem, and pars nervosa. Nerve fibres from the hypothalamic area of the brain grow into the pars nervosa.

The stalk of Rathke's pouch, which connects it to the stomodeum, normally degenerates and disappears in Week 6.

45. HYPOPHYSIS CEREBRI (PITUITARY GLAND)
STAGE 18   STAGE 18

DIENCEPHALON

TONGUE (Y)

(Y)

(O)

(Y)

floor of diencephalon —

neuro-hypophyseal bud (O)

(O)

(O)

Rathke's pouch (ℓG)

(Y)

(ℓG)

primordium of sphenoid bone (Y)

STAGE 19   STAGE 21

(O)

(O)

(ℓG)

(Y)

(Y)

neurohypophyseal bud (O)
(posterior lobe)

stalk of Rathke's pouch

Rathke's pouch (ℓG)
(anterior lobe)

(O)

(ℓG)

(O)

(O)

(Y)

(ℓG)

STAGE 23   ADULT

(O)

(O)

(ℓG)

(O)

(Y) (Y)

(ℓG)

pars tuberalis

pars distalis
(anterior lobe)

pars nervosa (O)
(posterior lobe)

(ℓG)

(O)

(Y)

(O)

pars nervosa (O)
(posterior lobe)

pars intermedia

(ℓG)

46. Special Senses: Eye

The eye develops from a combination of four types of tissue: neural ectoderm, surface ectoderm, mesoderm, and neural crest cells.

The eye is first evident in Week 4, when an optic sulcus appears on each unfused neural fold. After the neural folds fuse to form the neural tube, the sulci form optic vesicles which grow towards the overlying head ectoderm. The optic vesicles are connected to the diencephalon by the optic stalks. Each vesicle induces the overlying surface ectoderm to thicken and form the lens placode. Next the optic vesicles and the lens placode invaginate. As the optic vesicles then form a double-walled optic cup, the intraretinal space is reduced to a narrow slit and the optic stalks each develop a groove called the optic fissure. The hyaloid artery and vein develop in this fissure from mesenchyme, and they will supply the inner layer of the optic cup and the lens as it develops in the embryo and fetus. Later, the edges of the optic fissure will fuse to enclose the artery, vein and mesenchyme cells.

The lens placode first forms a lens pit and eventually a lens vesicle develops as it separates from the surface ectoderm.

Optic Cup

The two layers of the double-walled optic cup eventually meet and fuse loosely. Thus the intraretinal space is obliterated. The inner layer of the optic cup will form the neural retina and the outer layer the retinal pigment epithelium. The anterior part of the cup forms the nonvisual parts of the retina.

The proximal parts of the hyaloid artery and vein remain to form the central artery and vein of the adult retina. The distal portions of the hyaloid artery disappear by birth and the lens is then avascular.

Optic Nerve

Axons from the cells in the neural retina grow into the optic stalk toward the diencephalon and form the optic nerve. They become myelinated during the late fetal period and over the next 10 weeks of the neonatal period.

Lens Placode

The lens will form from the lens vesicle: the epithelium of the anterior wall of the vesicle forms the thin-layered anterior lens epithelium. The epithelium of the posterior wall of the vesicle enlarges and thickens greatly to form anucleate primary lens fibres. As this layer thickens, the lumen of the lens vesicle is obliterated. Anucleated secondary lens fibres differentiate at the equator of the lens from the epithelial cells and the diameter of the lens continues to increase in size.

Iris and Ciliary Body

The anterior part of the optic cup grows over the anterior part of the lens. It forms the epithelium of the iris and ciliary body and sphincter and dilator pupillae muscles of the iris. They are, therefore, neuroectodermal in origin, while mesenchyme around the rim of the optic cup forms the ciliary muscles and connective tissue. The iris is bluish in most neonates and the adult eye colour is acquired as pigment is laid down in the months after birth. The cells responsible for the pigmentation are neural crest derivatives.

46. SPECIAL SENSES: EYE

STAGE 13

optic vesicle

lens placode

ectoderm layer

(Y)
(O)
(O)

STAGE 14

lens placode (O)

intraretinal space

(Y)

(O)

hyaloid artery (dR)

STAGE 15

lens vesicle (O)

outer and inner layers of optic cup (Y)

ectoderm layer

(O)
(dR)

STAGE 17

(O)

lens (O)

hyaloid artery (dR)

STAGE 19

sclera (lG)

(Y) (Y)

(O)

(dR)

(Y)

(lG)

(O)

primordium of eyelid

WEEK 10

pigment epithelium and neural layer of the retina (Y)

choroid coat

sclera (lG)

fused eyelids (O)

anterior chamber

(O)

(dR)

conjunctival sac

hyaloid artery (dR)

Choroid, Sclera and Cornea

The optic cup and stalk are surrounded by mesenchyme cells which condense to form two layers. The inner layer forms the choroid layer of the eye and is continuous with the pia and arachnoid meninges. The outer layer forms the sclera of the eye and the substantia propria of the cornea and is continuous with the dura which surrounds the optic nerve and brain. These relationships are important clinically. A high pressure in the cerebrospinal fluid (CSF) results in papilloedema and can be detected by examining the eye.

Anteriorly the cornea is derived from the surface ectoderm.

Aqueous Chambers

Two separate aqueous chambers develop in the eye: an anterior chamber between the developing iris and cornea, and a posterior chamber between the developing iris and lens. These two chambers are separated by the pupillary membrane, a layer of connective tissue covering the pupil. In Week 20 this membrane degenerates as the pupil forms, and the two chambers are brought into communication.

Vitreous Body

As the optic cup forms, the surrounding mesenchyme enters the double-layered cup. This mesenchyme differentiates into part of the vitreous humor. Later there is a large contribution of vitreous humor which is formed from the inner wall of the optic cup.

Eyelids

Eyelids develop as the surface ectoderm and the underlying mesenchyme proliferate superior and inferior to the cornea. The glands and eyelashes form from the surface ectoderm and the tarsal plates and connective tissue differentiate from the mesenchyme.

The eyelids grow towards one another and fuse in Week 8. They remain closed during the period of retinal differentiation and reopen in Week 26.

Anomalies of the Eye

Failure of fusion of the optic fissure results in congenital coloboma. This may involve the iris or the retina.

Congenital cataract, resulting in blindness, may be the result of a maternal rubella virus infection (German measles).

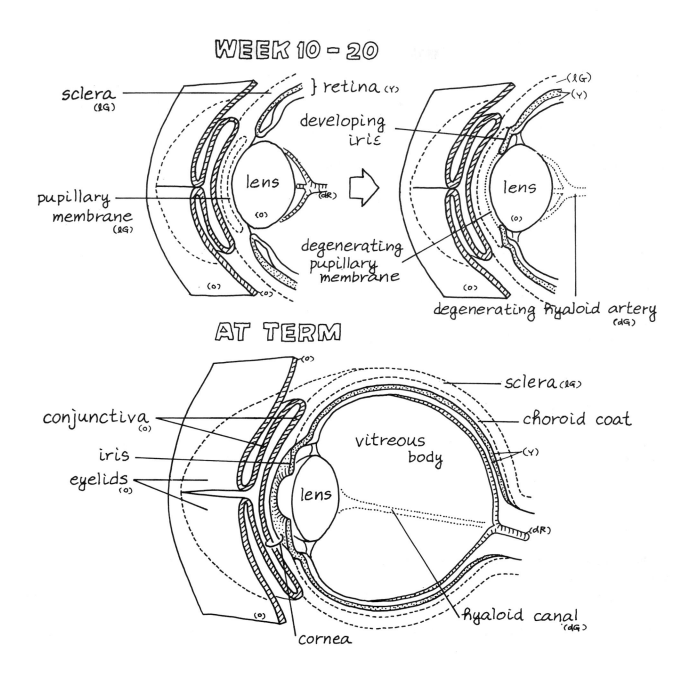

WEEK 10 - 20

sclera (ℓG)

} retina (Y)

developing iris

lens

pupillary membrane (ℓG)

(0)

(dR)

degenerating pupillary membrane

(ℓG)

(Y)

lens

(0)

(0)

degenerating hyaloid artery (dG)

AT TERM

(0)

conjunctiva (0)

sclera (ℓG)

choroid coat

iris

vitreous body

(Y)

eyelids (0)

lens

(dR)

cornea

(0)

hyaloid canal (dG)

47. Special Senses: Ear (Including External Ear)

The ear is divided into three major regions: the internal (inner) ear; the middle ear; and the external ear.

Internal Ear

In Week 4, the surface ectoderm thickens to form the otic placode which is found near the region of the hindbrain. The otic placode then invaginates to form an otic pit. As the otic pit loses its connection with the surface ectoderm, the edges of the pit fuse to form the otic vesicle (otocyst). The otic vesicle is the primordium of the membranous labyrinth. A tubular diverticulum from the otic vesicle develops and later forms the endolymphatic duct and sac.

The otic vesicle becomes constricted near its middle to form two major regions: a dorsal utricular portion and a ventral saccular portion. The derivatives of the utricular portion are the utricle, the endolymphatic duct and the three semicircular ducts. The saccular portion gives rise to the saccule and cochlear duct. The cochlear duct spirals to form the cochlea and the spiral organ (of Corti) differentiates in its walls.

47. SPECIAL SENSES: EAR
(INCLUDING EXTERNAL EAR)
INTERNAL EAR
STAGE 10

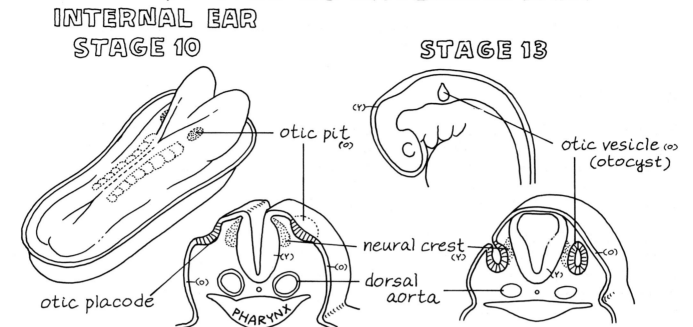

otic pit (O)

otic placode

neural crest (Y)

dorsal aorta

PHARYNX

STAGE 13

otic vesicle (O)
(otocyst)

STAGE 13   STAGE 16   STAGE 17

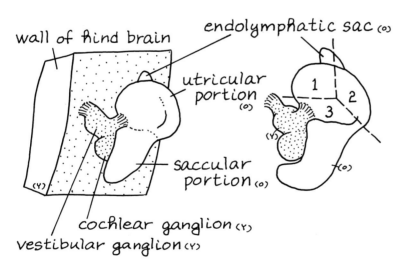

wall of hind brain

endolymphatic sac (O)

utricular portion (O)

saccular portion (O)

cochlear ganglion (Y)

vestibular ganglion (Y)

developing semicircular ducts (O)

developing cochlear duct

STAGE 23

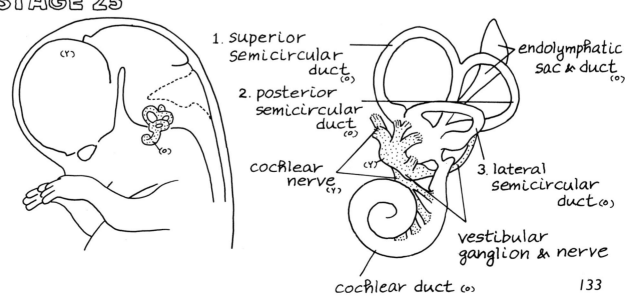

1. superior semicircular duct (O)

2. posterior semicircular duct (O)

cochlear nerve (Y)

endolymphatic sac & duct (O)

3. lateral semicircular duct (O)

vestibular ganglion & nerve

cochlear duct (O)

The Middle Ear

The first pharyngeal pouch extends and expands to form the tubotympanic recess which eventually envelopes the auditory ossicles (middle ear bones). The tympanic membrane forms where the recess contacts the ectoderm of the first branchial groove and its associated mesoderm.

The auditory ossicles derive from the cartilages of Branchial Arches I and II.

The proximal part of the tubotympanic recess forms the auditory tube while an extension of the tubotympanic recess forms the mastoid antrum. The mastoid process is not present at birth and the facial nerve is exposed to possible injury, e.g. during a forceps delivery. The mastoid process develops around 2 years of age.

The External Ear

The auricle develops from the six auricular hillocks around the dorsal end of the first branchial grooves. The hillocks fuse to form the auricle.

The external acoustic meatus is a derivative of the first branchial groove and is normally filled by the meatal plug until near birth.

Anomalies of the Ear

Maternal infection with the rubella virus may lead to congenital deafness.

MIDDLE AND EXTERNAL EAR

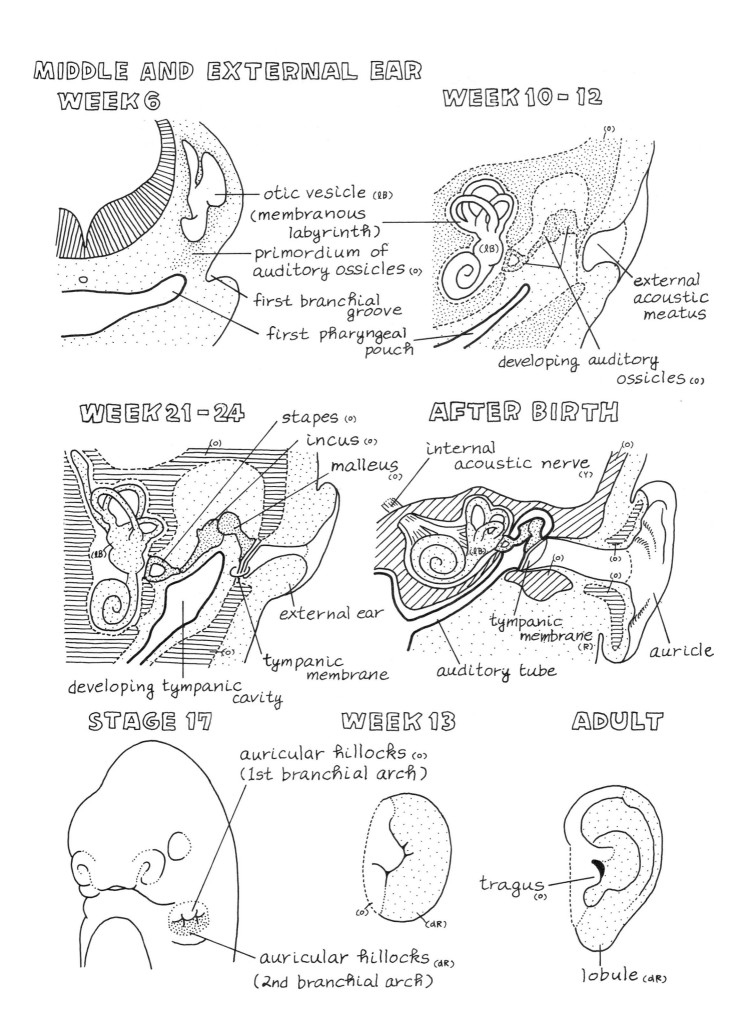

WEEK 6

otic vesicle (ℓB)
(membranous labyrinth)

primordium of auditory ossicles (o)

first branchial groove

first pharyngeal pouch

WEEK 10 - 12

external acoustic meatus

developing auditory ossicles (o)

WEEK 21 - 24

stapes (o)

incus (o)

malleus (o)

external ear

tympanic membrane

developing tympanic cavity

AFTER BIRTH

internal acoustic nerve (Y)

tympanic membrane (R)

auricle

auditory tube

STAGE 17

auricular hillocks (o)
(1st branchial arch)

auricular hillocks (dR)
(2nd branchial arch)

WEEK 13

ADULT

tragus (o)

lobule (dR)

48. Special Senses: Olfactory Nerve (I)

The epithelial lining of the nasal sac differentiates in the general area of the superior concha wall into bipolar neurons. The unmyelinated axons form the 18–20 bundles of the olfactory nerve (I). These bundles then pass superiorly and end in the olfactory bulb.

48. SPECIAL SENSES: OLFACTORY NERVE (I)
STAGE 15

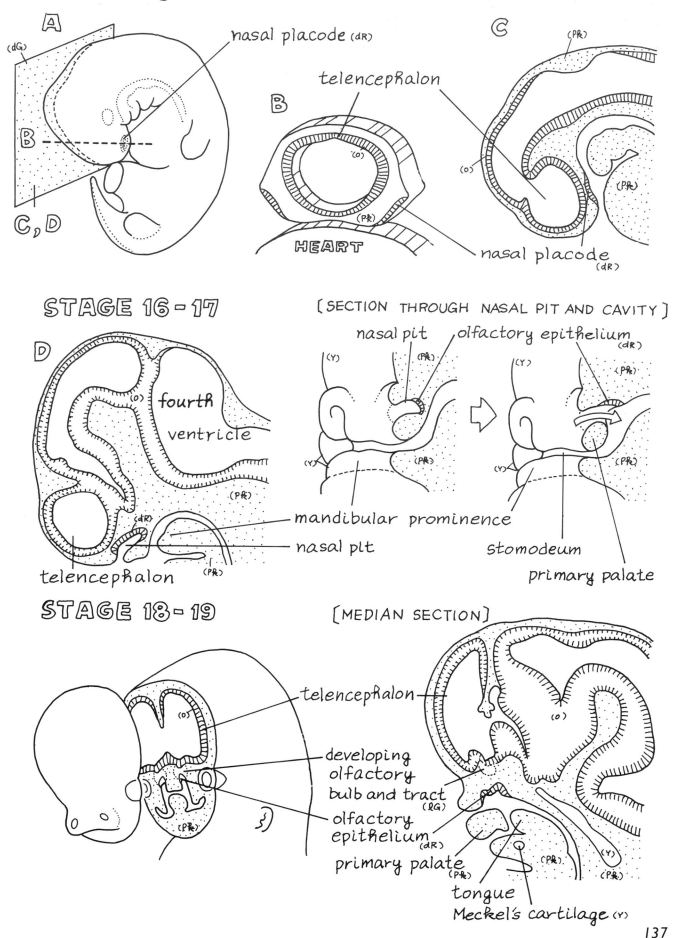

A (dG)

nasal placode (dR)

C (PR)

B telencephalon

B (o) (PR)

C (o) (PR)

HEART

nasal placode (dR)

STAGE 16 - 17

D (o) *fourth* *ventricle* (PR)

telencephalon (PR)

[SECTION THROUGH NASAL PIT AND CAVITY]

nasal pit olfactory epithelium (dR)

(Y) (PR) (Y) (PR)

(Y) (PR) (Y) (PR)

mandibular prominence

nasal pit

stomodeum

primary palate

STAGE 18 - 19

[MEDIAN SECTION]

telencephalon

(o) (o)

developing olfactory bulb and tract (lG)

olfactory epithelium (dR)

primary palate (PR)

(PR) (PR) (Y)

(PR)

tongue

Meckel's cartilage (Y)

As the olfactory bundles pass superiorly to the olfactory bulb, the cribriform plate of the ethmoid bone develops around the 18–20 bundles of axons of the olfactory cells.

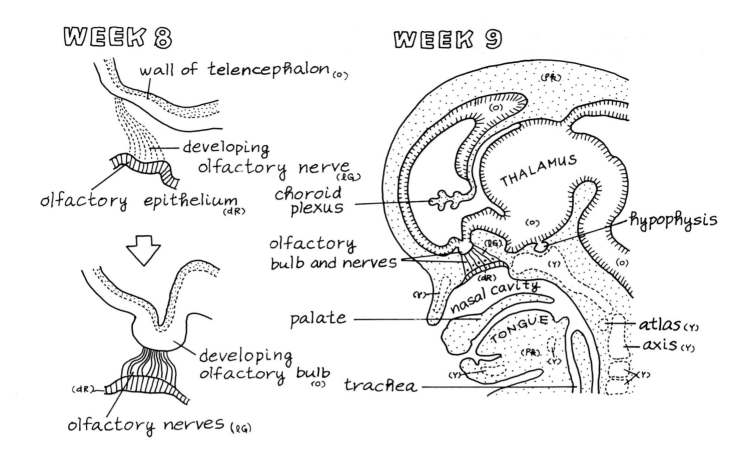

WEEK 8

wall of telencephalon (O)

developing olfactory nerve (ℓG)

olfactory epithelium (dR)

developing olfactory bulb (O)

(dR)

olfactory nerves (ℓG)

WEEK 9

(PR)

(O)

THALAMUS

choroid plexus

(O)

hypophysis

olfactory bulb and nerves

(ℓG)

(dR)

(Y)

nasal cavity

(Y)

(O)

palate

TONGUE

atlas (Y)

axis (Y)

(PR)

(Y)

(Y)

(Y)

trachea

(Y)

49. Peripheral Nervous System

Cranial Nerves

The cranial nerves develop in Weeks 5–6 and arise as three major groups.

a) Special Sensory Nerves

Cranial Nerve I (olfactory) is composed of the axons of bipolar neurons in the nasal olfactory epithelium. Between 18 and 20 bundles of axons grow into each olfactory bulb.

Cranial Nerve II (optic): fibres arise from neuroblasts in the retina which grow along the optic stalk. The optic nerve is really a pathway of the brain rather than a nerve.

Cranial Nerve VIII (vestibulocochlear) is composed of two nerves: the vestibular nerve and the cochlear nerve.

The vestibular nerve is composed of bipolar neurons whose cell bodies are in the vestibular ganglion. The peripheral processes originate in the semicircular ducts and the central processes terminate in the vestibular nuclei in the floor of the fourth ventricle.

The cochlear nerve is composed of bipolar neurons whose cell bodies are in the spiral ganglion. The peripheral processes originate in the spiral organ of Corti and central processes terminate in the ventral and dorsal cochlear nuclei in the medulla.

b) Somatic Efferent Nerves

These nerves are homologous with the ventral roots of the spinal nerves, and include the greater part of Cranial Nerve III (oculomotor), Cranial Nerve IV (trochlear), Cranial Nerve VI (abducens) and Cranial Nerve XII (hypoglossal). Their cells of origin lie in the basal plates (somatic efferent column) of the brainstem. Their axons supply the muscles derived from the preotic and occipital head myotomes.

c) Branchial Arch Nerves

The branchial arch nerves are Cranial Nerve V (trigeminal), Cranial Nerve VII (facial), Cranial Nerve IX (glossopharyngeal) and Cranial Nerve X (vagus) and supply the branchial arches.

Cranial Nerve V supplies Branchial Arch I; Cranial Nerve VII supplies Arch II; Cranial Nerve IX supplies Arch III, and Cranial Nerve X supplies the fused Arches IV and VI. They all innervate the derivatives of these arches.

Cranial Nerve XI (accessory) arises from an extension of Cranial Nerve X (a cranial root) and from the cranial five or six cervical segments of the spinal cord (spinal root).

49. PERIPHERAL NERVOUS SYSTEM

CRANIAL NERVES
STAGE 14

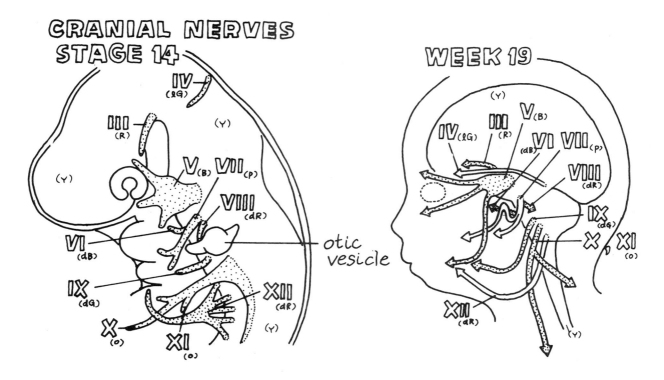

WEEK 19

otic vesicle

Autonomic Nervous System

The neural crest gives rise to Schwann cells, most of the autonomic nervous system and all the chromaffin tissue.

The autonomic nervous system is comprised of the sympathetic (thoracolumbar) and parasympathetic (craniosacral) systems.

Sympathetic System

The sympathetic nervous system arises in Week 5 when some of the thoracic neural crest cells migrate around the spinal cord and become located dorsolateral to the aorta. Here they form a chain of para-vertebral sympathetic ganglia connected by nerve fibres so forming the sympathetic trunks. Other neural crest cells migrate ventral to the aorta and contribute neurons to the preaortic ganglia. A further group of neural crest cells migrate to form terminal ganglia in sympathetic plexuses associated with the heart, lungs and gastrointestinal tract.

Following the basic formation of the sympathetic trunks, ascending and descending fibres are incorporated into the sympathetic chains.

Axons from sympathetic neurons in the lateral horn of the thoracolumbar spinal cord pass to each paravertebral ganglion via the ventral root of the spinal nerve and the white ramus communicans. There, some of the preganglionic fibres either ascend or descend in the sympathetic trunk to synapse at another level. Other axons enter and synapse directly at the same level. Some axons enter and pass through the paravertebral ganglia without synapsing to form splanchnic nerves which supply the viscera. Postganglionic fibres pass from a sympathetic ganglion through a grey ramus communicans into a spinal nerve.

Parasympathetic System

The parasympathetic nervous system is concerned with craniosacral elements. Preganglionic fibres originate in the brainstem nuclei of Cranial Nerves III, VII, IX and X and in the sacral spinal cord. Postganglionic neurons are located in plexuses or peripheral ganglia in close association with the structure being innervated (e.g. heart, pupil of eye).

Anomalies of the Peripheral Nervous System

Congenital aganglionic megacolon (Hirschsprung disease) is characterised by the failure of the neural crest to migrate into the colon wall and differentiate into parasympathetic ganglion cells. The absence of ganglion cells in the myenteric plexus (Auerbach's plexus) of the rectum/sigmoid colon results in faecal retention and abdominal distention.

AUTONOMIC NERVOUS SYSTEM
STAGE 13-14

from STAGE 19

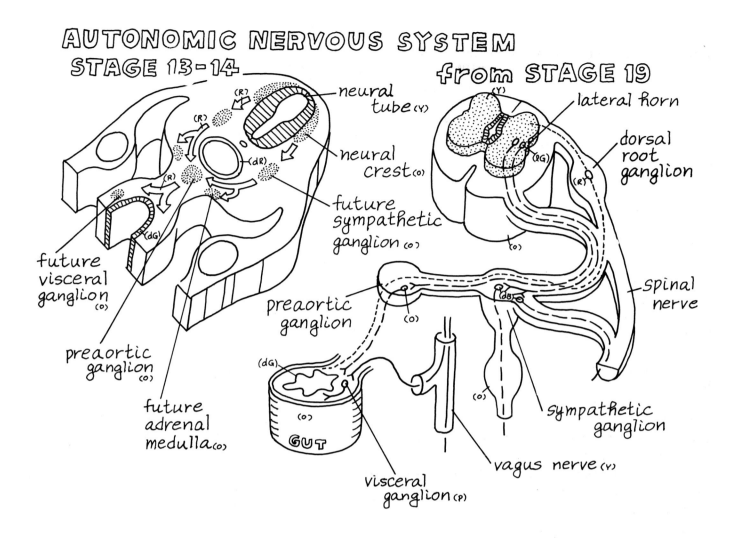

neural tube (V)

neural crest (O)

future sympathetic ganglion (O)

future visceral ganglion (O)

preaortic ganglion (O)

future adrenal medulla (O)

lateral horn

dorsal root ganglion

preaortic ganglion

spinal nerve

sympathetic ganglion

vagus nerve (V)

visceral ganglion (P)

GUT

BRANCHIAL APPARATUS

50. Branchial Arches

In the early embryo, a series of arches, pouches, grooves and membranes develops in the pharyngeal region of the head and neck. These structures are referred to as the branchial apparatus and superficially bear a resemblance to gills. They are transient structures which support the cranial foregut and they are then rearranged to form new structures or they disappear.

There are six branchial arches numbered I–VI in a craniocaudal order. Only the first four are visible externally. Externally the arches are separated from one another by branchial grooves. Each arch is composed of a core of mesenchymal cells. The external epithelial surface of each arch is a thin layer of ectoderm and their internal epithelial surface is endoderm lining the branchial arches. Internally pharyngeal pouches are present between the branchial arches. Here the lining endoderm and the surface ectoderm abut to form the branchial membranes.

The mesenchyme of each arch originates from the lateral mesoderm (see **13**. Derivatives of the Germ Layers: Mesoderm at the Somite Stage, p.47) and neural crest cells which have migrated into the arch. The mesenchyme will form cartilages, bones, muscles and blood vessels. The neural crest cells will give rise to some skeletal elements e.g. the maxilla. Cranial nerves will also grow into each arch from the brain. A typical branchial arch contains a cartilaginous bar, a muscular element, a cranial nerve supply and an artery.

Branchial Arch I is also known as the mandibular arch. It will give rise to two swellings: a cephalic one and a caudal one. The cephalic swelling, a small maxillary prominence, will form the maxilla (upper jaw), zygomatic bone, and the squamous part of the temporal bone. The caudal swelling, a larger mandibular prominence will develop into the mandible (lower jaw), malleus, incus and contribute to the auricle of the external ear (see **47**. Special Senses: Ear).

Branchial Arch II is also known as the hyoid arch because of its contribution to the hyoid bone.

The remaining arches are referred to only by their number. Arch V is frequently absent and if present lacks a cartilaginous bar. The cartilaginous bars of the Arches IV and VI fuse to form the laryngeal cartilages.

BRANCHIAL APPARATUS

50. BRANCHIAL ARCHES

STAGE 13

STAGE 13

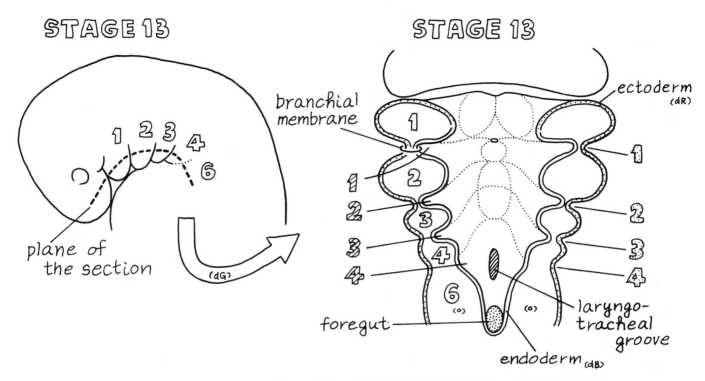

plane of the section

(dG)

branchial membrane

ectoderm (dR)

1

1

2

2

3

4

foregut

6 (o)

(o)

laryngo-tracheal groove

endoderm (dB)

1~6: BRANCHIAL ARCHES
1~4: PHARYNGEAL POUCHES
1~4: BRANCHIAL GROOVES

STAGE 13

STAGE 17

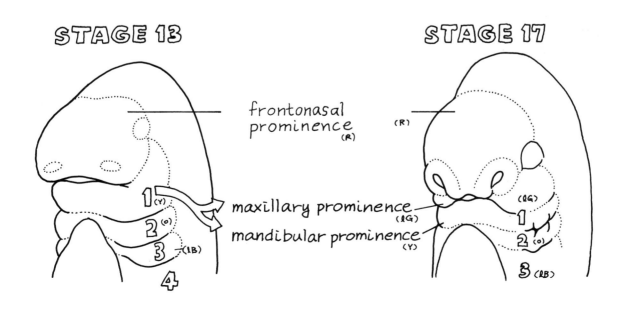

frontonasal prominence (R)

(R)

maxillary prominence (lG)

mandibular prominence (Y)

1 (Y)

2 (o)

3 (lB)

4

1 (lG)

2 (o)

3 (lB)

51. Derivatives of the Branchial Arches: Skeleton, Muscles, Arteries, Nerves and Other Tissues

Branchial Arch Skeleton

In each arch, except Arch V, mesenchyme and neural crest contributions condense to form a cartilaginous bar, the branchial arch cartilage.

Branchial Arch I

The majority (and ventral part) of the Arch I cartilage is referred to as Meckel's cartilage. It serves as scaffolding for the intramembranous development of the mandible. The dorsal end forms the middle ear bones the malleus and incus. The intermediate portion regresses and its perichondrium forms the anterior ligament of the malleus and the sphenomandibular ligament.

Branchial Arch II

The dorsal end of the second branchial arch is referred to as Reichert's cartilage. It will ossify to form the stapes (middle ear bone) and the styloid process of the temporal bone. The intermediate portion regresses and its perichondrium forms the stylohyoid ligament. The ventral end of this arch cartilage ossifies to form the superior part and lesser cornu of the hyoid bone.

Branchial Arch III

This cartilage forms the inferior part of the greater cornu and body of the hyoid bone.

Branchial Arches IV and VI

These cartilages fuse to form all of the laryngeal cartilages except the epiglottis (see **65**. Larynx).

Branchial Arch Muscles

Branchial Arch I

Muscles derived from Arch I include the muscles of mastication (medial and lateral pterygoids, masseter, temporalis), the mylohyoid, the anterior belly of the digastric muscle, the tensor tympani, and tensor veli palatini.

Branchial Arch II

The muscles derived from Arch II include the muscles of facial expression (frontalis, orbicularis oris, orbicularis oculi, auricularis, buccinator, platysma), the stapedius, the stylohyoid and the posterior belly of the digastric muscle.

Branchial Arch III

The Arch III muscle is stylopharyngeus.

Branchial Arches IV and VI

The muscles formed from Arches IV and VI are the striated muscles of the oesophagus, constrictors of the pharynx, intrinsic laryngeal muscles, levator veli palatini and the cricothyroid muscle.

51. DERIVATIVES OF THE BRANCHIAL ARCHES: SKELETON, MUSCLES, ARTERIES, NERVES AND OTHER TISSUES

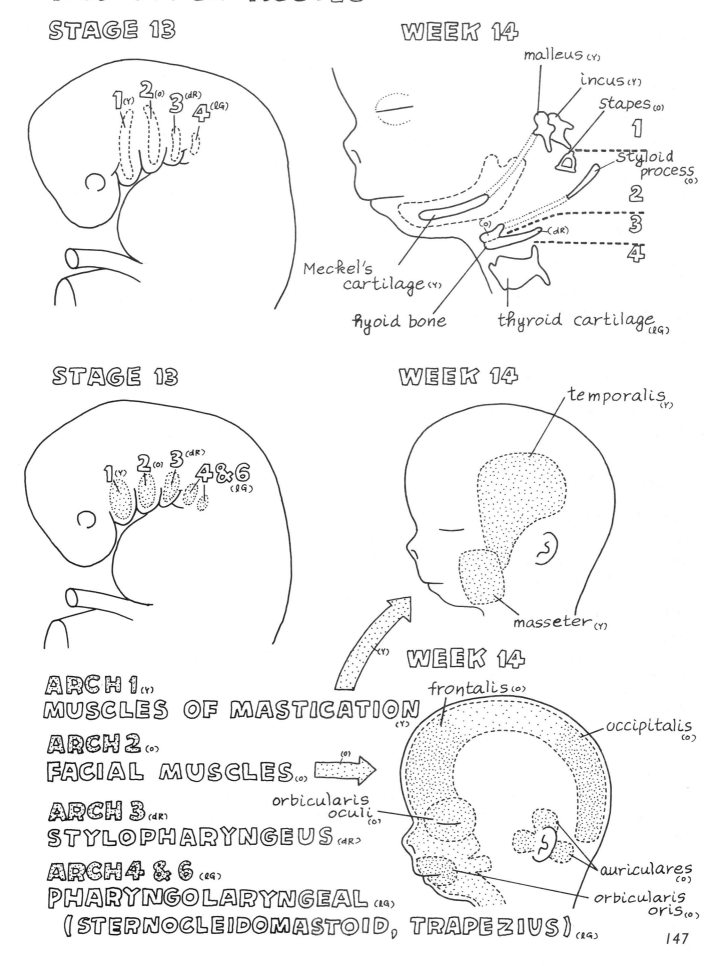

STAGE 13

WEEK 14

malleus (Y)
incus (Y)
stapes (O)
1
styloid process (O)
2
3
4
(O)
(dR)

Meckel's cartilage (Y)
hyoid bone
thyroid cartilage (LG)

STAGE 13

1 (Y) 2 (O) 3 (dR) 4 & 6 (LG)

WEEK 14

temporalis (Y)

masseter (Y)

WEEK 14

frontalis (O)
occipitalis (O)
orbicularis oculi (O)
auriculares (O)
orbicularis oris (O)

ARCH 1 (Y)
MUSCLES OF MASTICATION (Y)

ARCH 2 (O)
FACIAL MUSCLES (O)

ARCH 3 (dR)
STYLOPHARYNGEUS (dR)

ARCH 4 & 6 (LG)
PHARYNGOLARYNGEAL (LG)
(STERNOCLEIDOMASTOID, TRAPEZIUS) (LG)

147

Branchial Arch Arteries

Each branchial arch is supplied by an aortic arch artery which originates from the aortic sac of the heart and joins to a dorsal aorta.

The aortic arch arteries are not all present at the same time. As the most caudal ones (VI) develop, the most cephalic ones (I and II) degenerate apart from the parts which will contribute to the adult vessels.

Aortic Arch I arteries largely disappear but contribute to the maxillary arteries and possibly to the external carotid arteries.

Aortic Arch II arteries contribute to the stems of the stapedial arteries.

The proximal parts of the Aortic Arch III arteries form the common carotid arteries; the distal parts and the dorsal aortae form the internal carotid arteries. The left Aortic Arch IV artery becomes the distal part of the arch of the aorta. The aortic sac gives rise to the proximal part of the arch of the aorta.

The right Aortic Arch IV artery forms the proximal part of the right subclavian artery while its distal part forms from the right dorsal aorta and right VIIth intersegmental artery. The left subclavian artery comes from the left VIIth intersegmental artery without any contribution from any aortic arch.

The Aortic Arch V arteries are rudimentary or never form and have no derivatives.

The left Aortic Arch VI arteries contribute proximally to the left pulmonary artery and distally as the ductus arteriosus. The right Aortic Arch VI artery contributes proximally to the right pulmonary arteries and distally degenerates.

Branchial Arch Nerves

The branchial arch nerves are given below:

Branchial Arch I

The trigeminal (V) nerve, maxillary and mandibular divisions. The ophthalmic division does not supply branchial arch derivatives.

Branchial Arch II

Facial (VII) nerve.

Branchial Arch III

Glossopharyngeal (IX) nerve.

Branchial Arch IV

Superior laryngeal branch of the vagus (X) nerve.

Branchial Arch VI

The recurrent laryngeal branch of the vagus (X) nerve.

Branchial Arch Derivatives: Other Tissues

The first and second branchial arches contribute extensively to the neck, larynx, nasal cavities, mouth, face and external ears (auricles) and pharynx.

STAGE 13

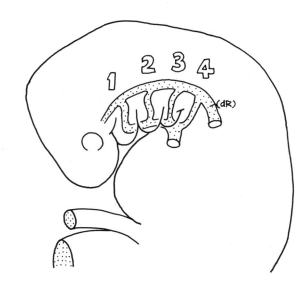

STAGE 18

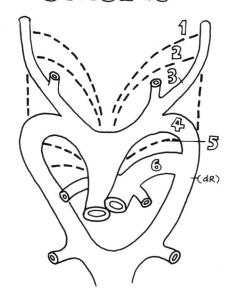

STAGE 13

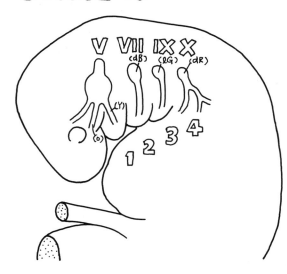

WEEK 14

▷ ARCH 1

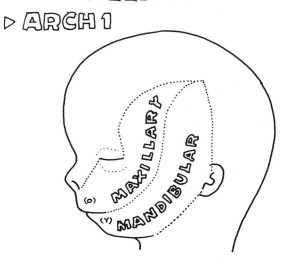

▷ ARCH 2, 3 and 4

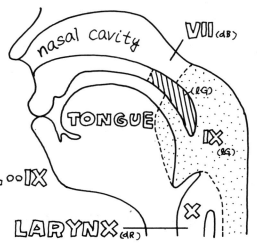

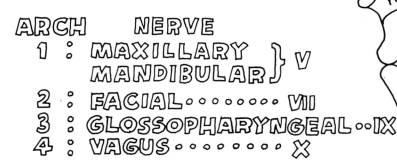

```
ARCH      NERVE
 1 : MAXILLARY   }
     MANDIBULAR  } V
 2 : FACIAL ∘∘∘∘∘∘∘ VII
 3 : GLOSSOPHARYNGEAL ∘∘ IX
 4 : VAGUS ∘∘∘∘∘∘∘∘ X
```

52. Pharyngeal Pouches and Branchial Grooves: Early

The four pharyngeal pouches are the endoderm-lined outpocketings of the pharynx. A fifth pair is atypical and is considered as part of the fourth pair. The pouches are numbered in a cranial to caudal sequence from 1 to 4 with the first pouch lying between Branchial Arches I and II. Where the pouches contact the ectodermal branchial grooves, the two layers together form the branchial membrane.

Externally, the first four branchial arches are separated by branchial grooves which are numbered in the same way as the pouches from 1 to 4. The first groove deepens and it contributes to the external acoustic meatus; its epithelial covering contributes to the formation of the eardrum.

Mesoderm in the second arch proliferates rapidly. By Stage 16, this arch grows caudally and overlays Arches III and IV and the 2, 3 and 4 branchial grooves. As Arch II fuses with Arch VI, the Arches III and IV and their grooves are buried, as is the space external to and adjacent to the arches. This space is called the cervical sinus and normally disappears with further growth and development. Grooves 2, 3 and 4 do not give rise to definitive structures.

52. PHARYNGEAL POUCHES AND BRANCHIAL GROOVES: EARLY

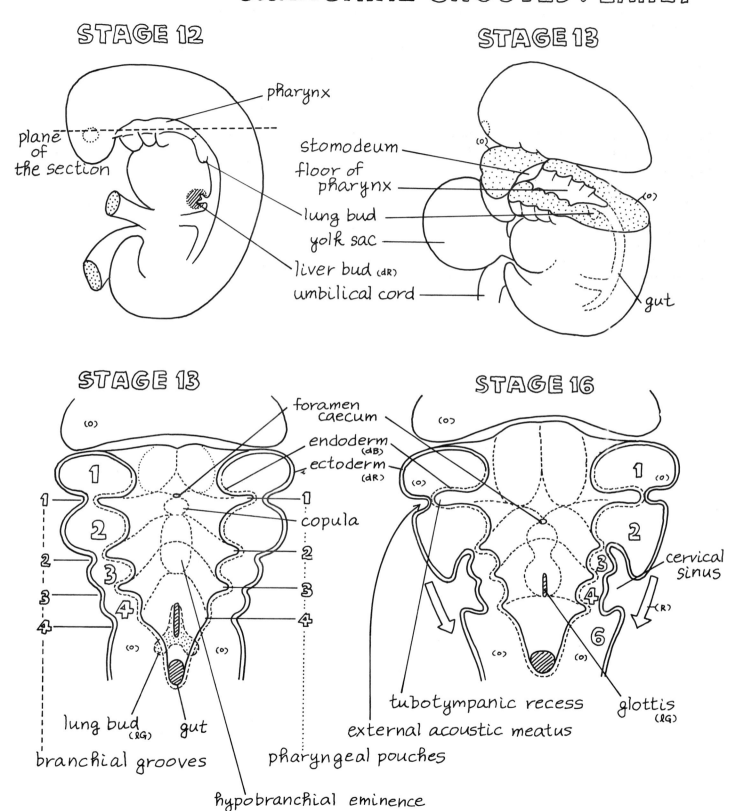

STAGE 12

plane
of
the section

pharynx

liver bud (dR)

STAGE 13

(o)

stomodeum
floor of
pharynx
lung bud
yolk sac
umbilical cord

gut

(o)

(o)

STAGE 13

(o)

1
2
3
4

1
2
3
4

foramen
caecum
endoderm
(dB)
ectoderm
(dR)

1
copula
2
3
4

lung bud
(lG)
gut

branchial grooves

pharyngeal pouches

hypobranchial eminence

STAGE 16

(o)

(o)

(o)

1
(o)

2

3
4

6

cervical
sinus

(R)

(o)
(o)

tubotympanic recess
external acoustic meatus

glottis
(lG)

151

53. Pharyngeal Pouches and their Derivatives

In the pharyngeal part of the foregut, the branchial arches are lined by endoderm and separated from one another by pharyngeal pouches. There are four distinct pouches and the fifth is rudimentary or absent.

Pharyngeal Pouch I

This pouch enlarges to form the tubotympanic recess which develops into the tympanic cavity and mastoid antrum. Its connection with the pharynx elongates to form the auditory (Eustachian) tube. The expanded distal portion of the pouch contacts the first branchial groove and contributes to the tympanic membrane (eardrum).

Pharyngeal Pouch II

The endodermal lining of Pouch II grows into the adjacent mesenchyme, and together they form the palatine tonsil. The mesenchyme forms lymphoid tissue and the endoderm forms the surface and crypt epithelia.

As the palatine tonsil develops, the pharyngeal pouch largely disappears. The remaining part forms the intratonsillar cleft.

Pharyngeal Pouch III

The endoderm lining the dorsal part of the pouch gives rise to the inferior parathyroid glands. The ventral part of the pouch gives rise to the thymus gland.

Pharyngeal Pouch IV

The endoderm lining the dorsal part of the pouch gives rise to the superior parathyroid glands. The ventral part of the pouch gives rise to the ultimobranchial bodies.

Anomalies of the Branchial Apparatus

Persistence of the cervical sinus may result in a branchial cyst. These cysts are usually present along the anterior border of the sternocleidomastoid muscle. If the sinus is connected to the external surface, it is referred to as a branchial sinus.

The first arch syndrome is believed to result from the incomplete migration of neural crest cells into the first branchial arch. There are various anomalies of the ears, eyes, mandible and palate. Two types of first arch syndrome are: the Treacher Collins syndrome (malformed ears and lower eyelids, and malar hypoplasia); and Pierre Robin syndrome (cleft palate, small mandible, ear and eye defects).

53. PHARYNGEAL POUCHES AND THEIR DERIVATIVES

STAGE 13

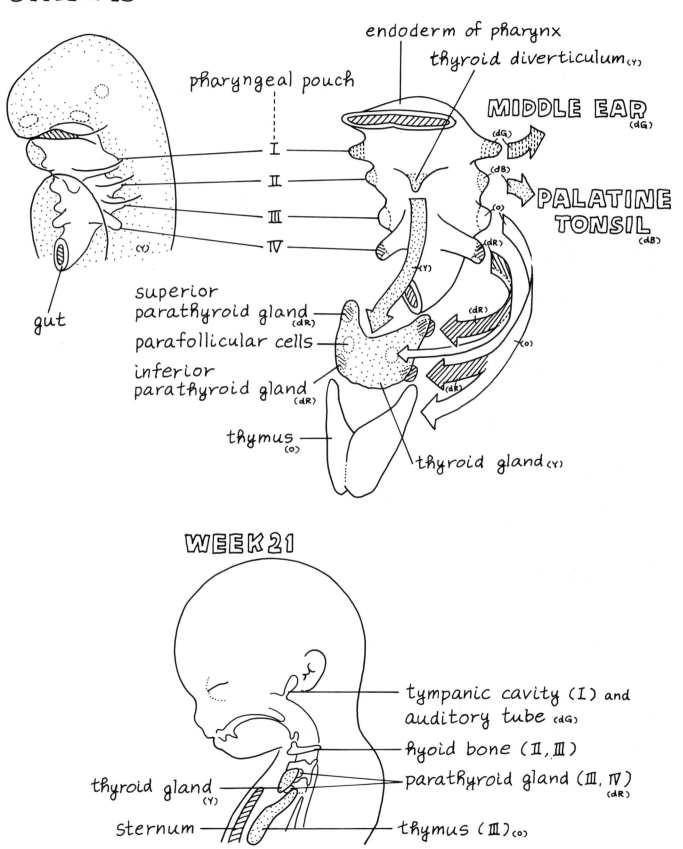

endoderm of pharynx

thyroid diverticulum (Y)

pharyngeal pouch

MIDDLE EAR (dG)

I

II (dB)

III (o)

IV (dR)

(Y)

PALATINE TONSIL (dB)

gut

(Y)

superior parathyroid gland (dR)

parafollicular cells

inferior parathyroid gland (dR)

(dR)

(o)

(dR)

thymus (o)

thyroid gland (Y)

WEEK 21

tympanic cavity (I) and auditory tube (dG)

hyoid bone (II, III)

parathyroid gland (III, IV) (dR)

thyroid gland (Y)

sternum

thymus (III) (o)

153

54. Development of the Tongue

The anterior two-thirds (body) of the tongue develops from three regions of the floor of the pharynx: the two distal tongue buds (lateral lingual swellings), and the single median tongue bud (tuberculum impar). These buds are derivatives of Branchial Arches I. The two lateral lingual swellings enlarge and fuse in the midline, and their line of fusion is marked in the adult by the median sulcus and septum. After fusion the swellings then grow over the median tongue bud.

The posterior one-third (root) of the tongue forms from the copula (ventromedial ends of Arch II) and hypobranchial eminence (Arch III and IV mesoderm). With growth, the hypobranchial eminence overgrows the copula. The anterior two-thirds and posterior one-third meet at a line approximately in the position of the 'V' shaped terminal sulcus region of the adult tongue. The taste buds develop in Weeks 7–9.

The sensory nerve supply of the mucous membrane of the anterior two-thirds (oral tongue) is the lingual nerve (including taste fibres from chorda tympani). The posterior one-third mucous membrane (pharyngeal tongue) is supplied by the glossopharyngeal nerve. The superior laryngeal nerve supplies a small area of mucous membrane adjacent to the epiglottis. The muscles mainly originate from occipital myotomes and are supplied by the hypoglossal nerve.

Anomalies of Tongue Development

Malformations of the tongue are uncommon. An excessively large tongue (macroglossia), an excessively small one (microglossia), or a bifid tongue are rare.

A frenulum extending to the tip of the inferior surface of the tongue (tongue tie) frequently corrects naturally as the infant grows.

54. DEVELOPMENT OF THE TONGUE

STAGE 13

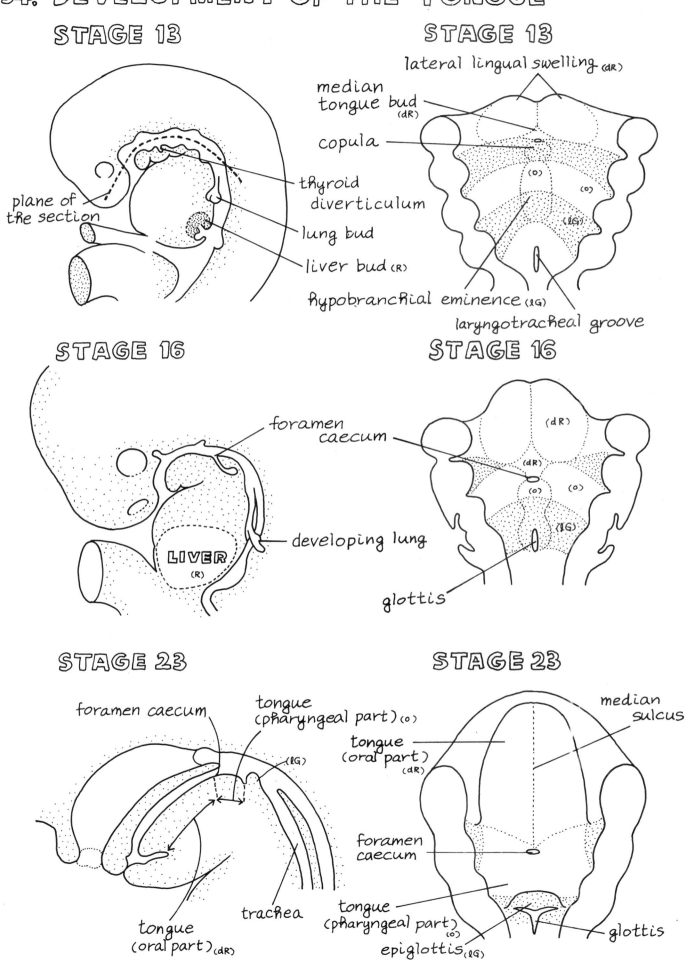

plane of the section

thyroid diverticulum

lung bud

liver bud (R)

STAGE 13

lateral lingual swelling (dR)

median tongue bud (dR)

copula

(o)

(o)

(lG)

hypobranchial eminence (lG)

laryngotracheal groove

STAGE 16

foramen caecum

LIVER (R)

developing lung

STAGE 16

(dR)

(dR)

(o)

(o)

(lG)

glottis

STAGE 23

foramen caecum

tongue (pharyngeal part) (o)

(lG)

trachea

tongue (oral part) (dR)

STAGE 23

median sulcus

tongue (oral part) (dR)

foramen caecum

tongue (pharyngeal part) (o)

epiglottis (lG)

glottis

155

55. Development of the Thyroid

The thyroid gland develops (Weeks 3–4) from the floor of the pharynx where the tongue will later develop. It forms as a downgrowth which descends into the neck forming a bilobed gland. For a period it retains contact with the back of the tongue via the thyroglossal duct. A pyramidal lobe may also form superior to the isthmus. This represents a persistent portion of the thyroglossal duct. This duct disappears (Week 7) but the position of its former opening is seen as the foramen caecum of the adult tongue.

The ultimobranchial body arises from the fourth pharyngeal pouch and fuses with the thyroid gland. It will give rise to the parafollicular or 'C' cells which produce calcitonin. The amine precursor uptake and decarboxylation (APUD) series of cells including the 'C' cells are neural crest derivatives.

55. DEVELOPMENT OF THE THYROID

STAGE 13

STAGE 16

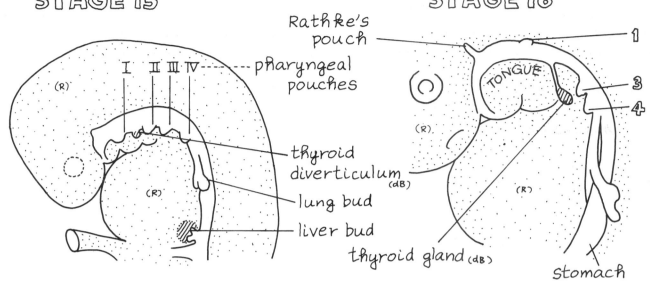

Rathke's pouch

pharyngeal pouches

I II III IV

(R)

thyroid diverticulum (dB)

lung bud

liver bud

(R)

1

3

4

TONGUE

(R)

(R)

thyroid gland (dB)

Stomach

STAGE 19

STAGE 23

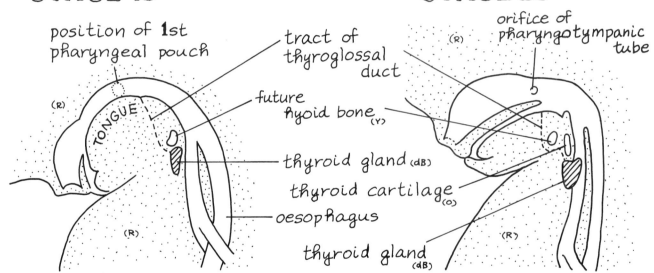

position of 1st pharyngeal pouch

(R)

TONGUE

(R)

tract of thyroglossal duct

future hyoid bone (Y)

thyroid gland (dB)

thyroid cartilage (O)

oesophagus

orifice of pharyngotympanic tube

(R)

(R)

thyroid gland (dB)

WEEK 10

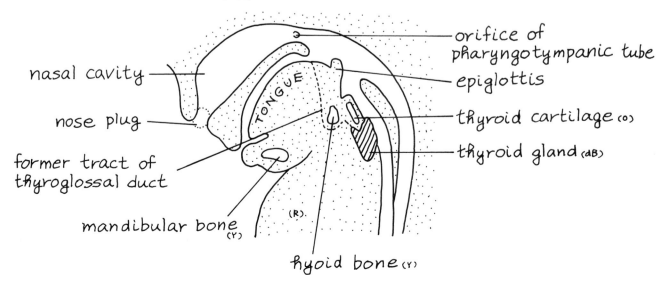

nasal cavity

nose plug

former tract of thyroglossal duct

mandibular bone (Y)

TONGUE

(R)

hyoid bone (Y)

orifice of pharyngotympanic tube

epiglottis

thyroid cartilage (O)

thyroid gland (dB)

The thyroid gland normally descends in the neck by passing ventral to the hyoid bone and the laryngeal cartilages.

Between Weeks 9 and 10 the endoderm of the gland forms epithelial plates as it is infiltrated by vascular mesenchyme. By Week 10 in the precolloid stage, the plates form small cell clusters each of which develops a lumen. The following week, colloid begins to form and iodide is concentrated in the thyroid follicle. By Week 14 thyroxine can be demonstrated.

Anomalies of Thyroid Development

Persistent remnants of the thyroglossal duct may give rise to cysts, sinuses or accessory thyroid tissue. A deficiency of fetal thyroid hormone results in cretinism. This is characterised by mental deficiency, auditory, neurological and skeletal abnormalities.

ADULT

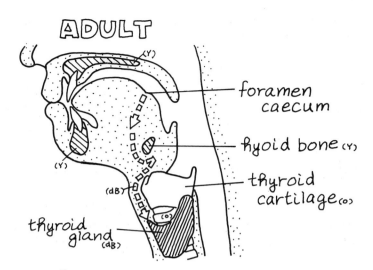

- foramen caecum
- hyoid bone (Y)
- thyroid cartilage (O)
- thyroid gland (dB)

HISTOLOGY OF THE THYROID GLAND

WEEK 9   WEEK 10   WEEK 14

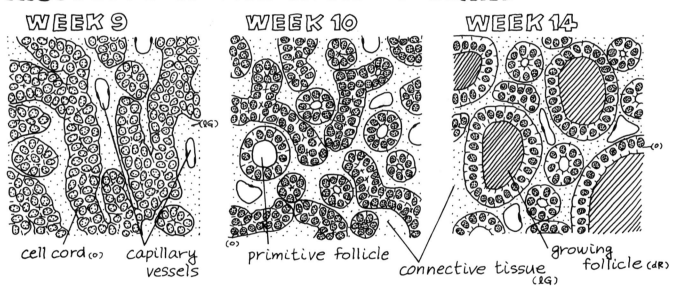

cell cord (O)   capillary vessels

primitive follicle

connective tissue (lG)

growing follicle (dR)

56. Development of the Parathyroid

The inferior parathyroid glands are derivatives of the dorsal part of Pharyngeal Pouch III (see **57.** Development of the Thymus). The superior parathyroid glands are derivatives of the dorsal part of Pharyngeal Pouch IV.

Both the superior IV and the inferior III parathyroid glands lie in the adult on the dorsal surface of the thyroid gland.

The superior parathyroid glands form in Week 6 from the endodermal dorsal portion of the Pharyngeal Pouch IV. The ventral elongated portion of this pouch will form the ultimobranchial body. Both the dorsal and ventral portions of Pouch IV are pinched off from the pharynx. The superior parathyroids fuse with and lie on the dorsal surface of the thyroid gland.

The inferior parathyroid glands migrate with the thymus and are carried caudal to the superior parathyroid glands before they separate from the thymus.

The ultimobranchial body is described in section **55.** Development of the Thyroid.

Anomalies of Parathyroid Development

Ectopic parathyroid glands may be found near or in the thymus or thyroid glands.

In Di George syndrome, Pharyngeal Pouches III and IV fail to differentiate into the parathyroid glands and thymus gland. Numerous other anomalies are present, including abnormalities of the mouth, ears, nose, heart and thyroid.

56. DEVELOPMENT OF THE PARATHYROID

STAGE 13

STAGE 17

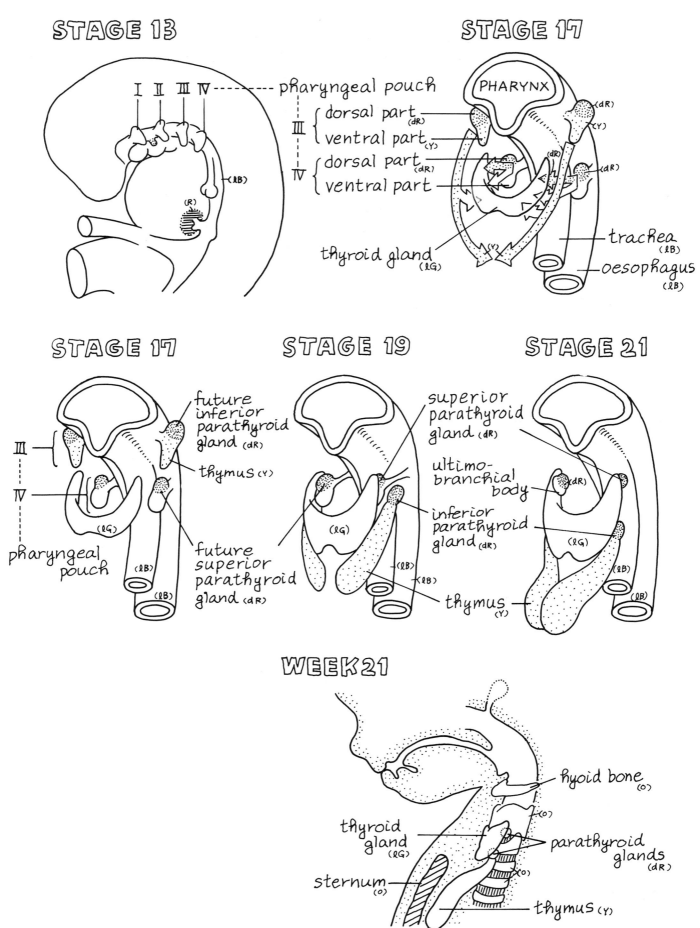

pharyngeal pouch

III { dorsal part (dR)
     ventral part (Y)

IV { dorsal part (dR)
     ventral part

PHARYNX

(dR)

(Y)

(dR)

(dR)

thyroid gland (ℓG)

trachea (ℓB)

oesophagus (ℓB)

STAGE 17

III

IV

pharyngeal pouch

future inferior parathyroid gland (dR)

thymus (Y)

future superior parathyroid gland (dR)

STAGE 19

superior parathyroid gland (dR)

ultimo-branchial body

inferior parathyroid gland (dR)

thymus (Y)

STAGE 21

(dR)

WEEK 21

hyoid bone (O)

(O)

thyroid gland (ℓG)

parathyroid glands (dR)

sternum (O)

(O)

thymus (Y)

161

57. Development of the Thymus

In Week 6, the dorsal and ventral parts of endodermal Pharyngeal Pouch III pinch off together from the pharynx. These two parts will initially migrate together. The dorsal portion will form the inferior parathyroid (III) glands and the hollow ventral portion will form the thymus.

In Weeks 7–8 the thymic primordia, one on each side elongate and migrate caudally. The inferior parathyroids are carried caudally with the thymic primordia and at the end of their migration, the inferior parathyroids come to lie on the dorsal surface of the thyroid gland in Week 7. They separate from the thymic primordia in Week 8 or slightly later.

As the thymic epithelium proliferates, the hollow in the primordium is obliterated. By Week 8 the two thymic primordia migrate medially and fuse. Hassall's corpuscles form from epithelium from the endoderm, while mesenchyme forms the septa. By Week 9 lymphocytes appear in this tissue.

The thymus in the neonate is variable in shape and may have no lobulation, be bilobar or trilobar. It is necessary for the development of the white pulp of the spleen and is important in the immunological development of the infant.

Anomalies of the Thymus

As the thymus migrates, portions of its trailing edge normally disintegrate and disappear. If these fragments persist, however, they may form isolated nests of thymic tissue or be embedded in the thyroid gland.

In Di George syndrome the thymus fails to develop.

57. DEVELOPMENT OF THE THYMUS

STAGE 17

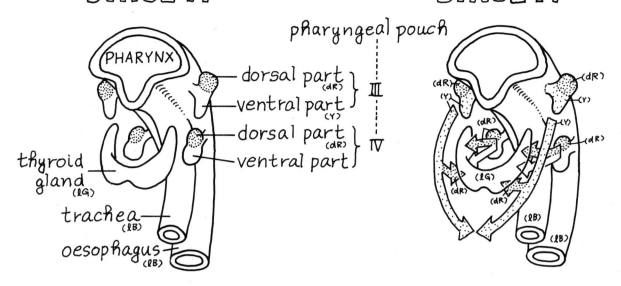

PHARYNX

pharyngeal pouch

dorsal part (dR) ⎫
ventral part (Y) ⎬ III

dorsal part (dR) ⎫
ventral part ⎬ IV

thyroid gland (lG)

trachea (lB)

oesophagus (lB)

STAGE 17

(dR)
(Y)
(dR)
(Y)
(dR)
(dR)
(lG)
(dR)
(lB)
(lB)

STAGE 19

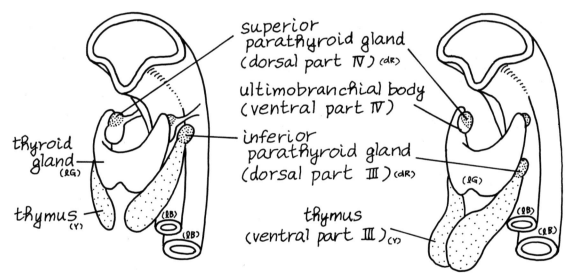

thyroid gland (lG)

thymus (Y)

(lB)
(lB)

superior parathyroid gland (dorsal part IV) (dR)

ultimobranchial body (ventral part IV)

inferior parathyroid gland (dorsal part III) (dR)

STAGE 21

thymus (ventral part III) (Y)

(lG)
(lB)
(lB)

WEEK 21

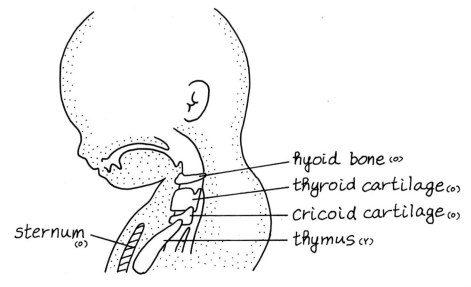

hyoid bone (O)

thyroid cartilage (O)

cricoid cartilage (O)

thymus (Y)

sternum (O)

58. Development of the Face

The face develops between Weeks 4–16 from five primordia. These are present in an area both bilateral and medial to the face region. The general movement of the bilateral elements is toward the midline of the face.

The five primordia circumscribe the stomodeum or primitive mouth. The frontonasal prominence (swelling) lies cranial to the primitive mouth (stomodeum); the lateral boundaries are formed by the two maxillary prominences (Branchial Arch I); and the caudal boundary is formed by the two paired and fused mandibular prominences (Branchial Arch I). The underlying mesenchyme of all five primordia is continuous and does not show the boundaries present on the surface.

The first elements to meet and fuse in the midline are the paired mandibular prominences in Week 4. They will form the lower lip, chin and mandible.

The medial frontonasal prominence will form the adult forehead, dorsum and tip of the nose. The frontonasal prominence develops two ectodermal surface thickenings, the nasal placodes. Ridges form around the depressed nasal placodes (nasal pits), called the medial and lateral nasal prominences.

The maxillary prominences will form the lateral parts of the upper lip, most of the maxilla and the secondary palate. In Weeks 5–8, the maxillary prominences increase in size, and the medial nasal prominences move medially and merge to form the intermaxillary segment which includes the nasal septum.

The intermaxillary segment is composed of three parts: a labial (lip) component which will form the philtrum of the upper lip; a palatal component (the primary palate); and a premaxillary component which will incorporate the four upper incisor teeth and their associated gum.

The lateral nasal prominences form the alae of the nose and do not form part of the upper lip. The line where the lateral nasal prominences meet the maxillary prominences is called the nasolacrimal groove.

Some of the mesenchyme from the first branchial arches forms the muscles of mastication which are supplied by the first arch nerve (V, trigeminal nerve). The skin covering this area is also supplied by V. Mesenchyme from the second arch invades the lips and cheeks to form the muscles of facial expression supplied by the second branchial arch nerve (VII, facial nerve).

The mouth develops from the stomodeum or primitive mouth, which is a depression in the surface ectoderm. The oropharyngeal membrane, which is composed of ectoderm externally and endoderm internally, ruptures at about 24–26 days. A direct communication is now established between the gut and the amniotic cavity.

58. DEVELOPMENT OF THE FACE

STAGE 13

STAGE 17

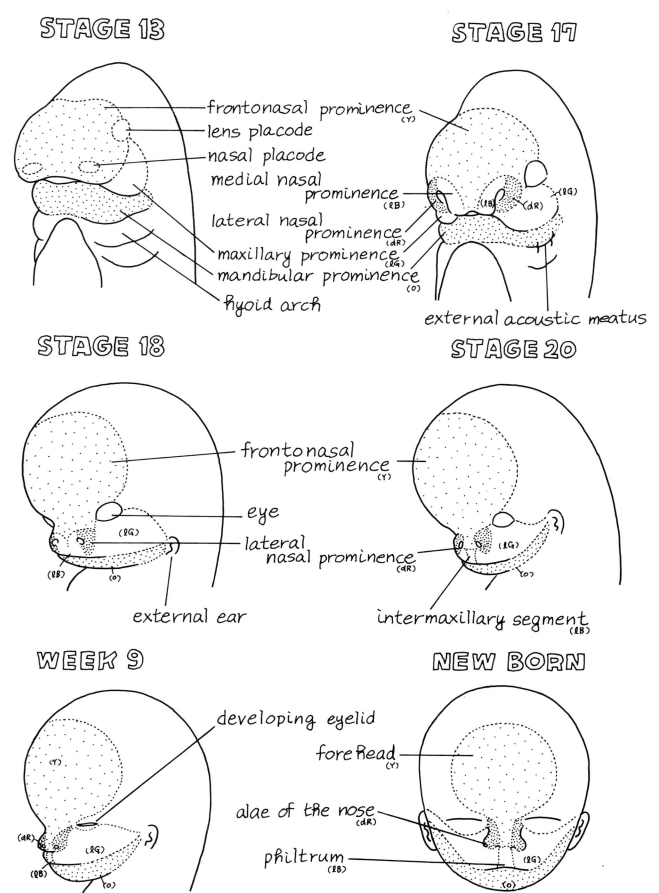

frontonasal prominence (Y)
lens placode
nasal placode
medial nasal prominence (ℓB)
lateral nasal prominence (dR)
maxillary prominence (ℓG)
mandibular prominence (o)
hyoid arch

external acoustic meatus

STAGE 18

STAGE 20

frontonasal prominence (Y)
eye
lateral nasal prominence (dR)
external ear

intermaxillary segment (ℓB)

WEEK 9

NEW BORN

developing eyelid
forehead (Y)
alae of the nose (dR)
philtrum (ℓB)

59. Development of the Palate

Formation of the palate is one of the last major morphogenetic events to occur (Weeks 5–12) in the embryo and fetus. It develops from three primordia: the median palatine process (or primary palate), and two lateral palatine processes.

Originally the lateral palatine processes project vertically on each side of the tongue. In Week 7, these processes move to a horizontal position above the tongue. The wedge-shaped median palatine process fuses in the median plane with the two shelf-like lateral palatine processes and with the inferior border of the nasal septum to form the secondary palate. (The nasal septum formed as a downgrowth from the fused medial nasal prominences.)

The position of the incisive foramen in the adult marks the point of fusion between the median palatine process and the two lateral palatine processes in the fetus. The foramen also serves as a landmark between the anterior and the posterior palates.

Bone gradually develops in the primary palate, forming the premaxillary part of the maxilla. Bone formation in the anterior portion of the fused lateral palatine processes creates the hard palate. The palate posterior to the hard palate forms the soft palate and uvula.

59. DEVELOPMENT OF THE PALATE
STAGE 16   STAGE 16-17

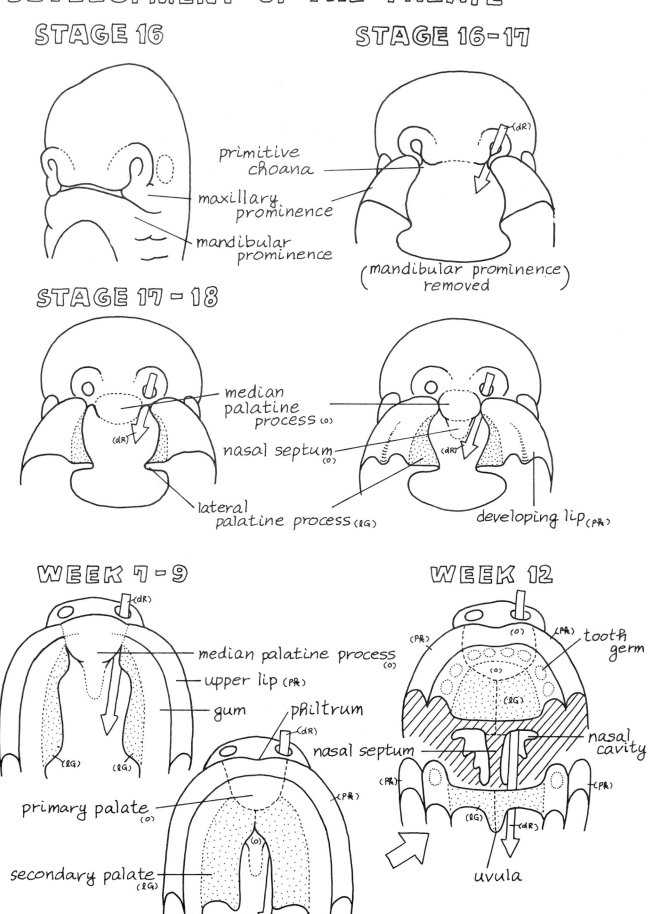

primitive
choana

maxillary
prominence

mandibular
prominence

(mandibular prominence)
removed

STAGE 17 - 18

median
palatine
process (o)

nasal septum
(o)

lateral
palatine process (lG)

developing lip (PR)

WEEK 7 - 9   WEEK 12

median palatine process
(o)

upper lip (PR)

gum

philtrum

tooth
germ

nasal septum

nasal
cavity

primary palate
(o)

secondary palate
(lG)

uvula

60. Cleft Lip and Cleft Palate

Cleft lip and cleft palate occurring either together or separately are the most commonly occurring defects of the face. They may occur as the result of either genetic inheritance or non-genetic (environmental) factors, and their frequency varies with ethnic origin.

Cleft lip occurs when the mesenchyme of the intermaxillary segment (medial nasal prominences) fails to merge with the maxillary prominence. This condition may be unilateral or bilateral, and may or may not be associated with the cleft palate.

Cleft palate refers to the failure of fusion of the hard and/or soft lateral palatine processes with each other and/or the nasal septum and/or the median palatine process. These clefts may be unilateral or bilateral.

Both the nerve supply and the positioning of the teeth are affected by anomalies of the lip or palate. Speech may be affected by these anomalies.

60. CLEFT LIP AND CLEFT PALATE

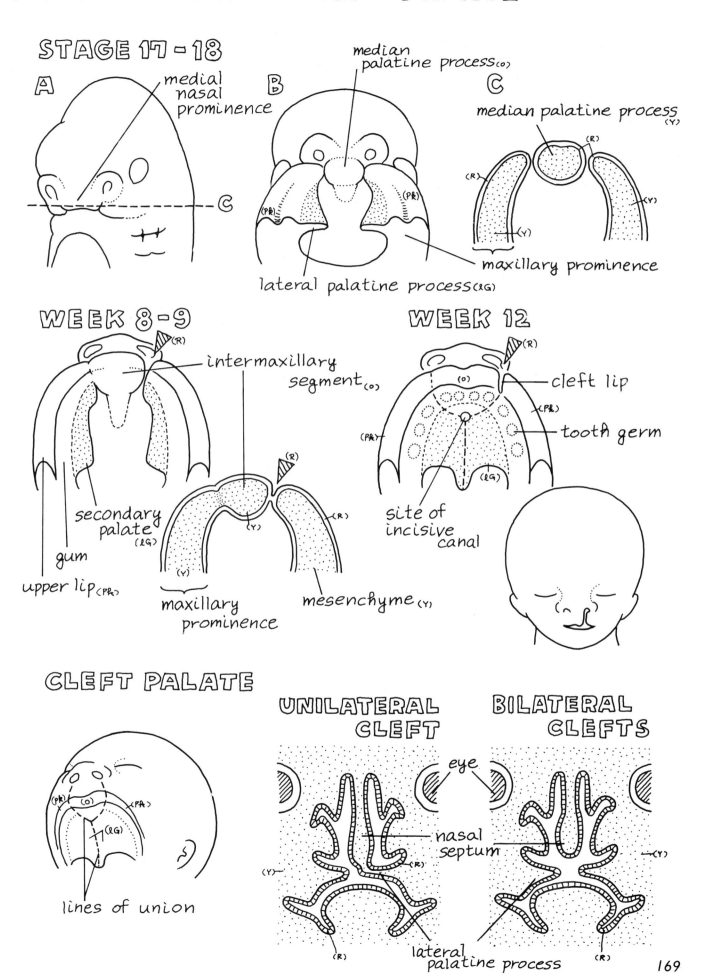

STAGE 17-18

A
medial nasal prominence

B
median palatine process(o)
lateral palatine process(ℓG)
maxillary prominence

C
median palatine process(Y)
(R)
(R)
(Y)
(Y)
maxillary prominence

WEEK 8-9

(R)
intermaxillary segment(o)
secondary palate(ℓG)
gum
upper lip(PR)
(R)
(Y)
maxillary prominence
(Y)
(R)
mesenchyme(Y)

WEEK 12

(R)
(O)
cleft lip
(PR)
tooth germ
(PR)
(ℓG)
site of incisive canal

CLEFT PALATE

(PR)
(O)
(PR)
(ℓG)
lines of union

UNILATERAL CLEFT

eye
nasal septum
(Y)
(R)
(R)

BILATERAL CLEFTS

eye
(Y)
lateral palatine process
(R)

169

DIVISION OF THE COELOM

61. Pleuropericardial Membranes

The intraembryonic coelom extends through the thoracic and abdominal regions. There is a single cavity in the thoracic region which will form the pericardial cavity. Two pericardioperitoneal canals connect this cavity with the abdominal cavity. Finally, the abdominal cavity is continuous with the extraembryonic coelom at the region of the umbilicus.

The division of the intraembryonic coelom into the pericardial cavity, pleural cavities and abdominal cavity occurs with the formation of the pleuropericardial membranes and diaphragm (see **62**. Diaphragm (Including Pleuroperitoneal Membranes) Formation).

The separation between the pleural (lung) cavities and the pericardial (heart) cavity occurs as the lungs grow into the pericardioperitoneal canals. A pair of bilateral ridges appear: a cephalic pleuropericardial membrane and a caudal pleuroperitoneal membrane. The former is superior to the lungs, and the latter inferior to the lungs. The cephalic pleuropericardial membrane on each side will enlarge and eventually the two membranes will meet and fuse in the midline. This separates the pericardial and pleural cavities. The detail of the process is as follows. Initially the membranes appear as ridges of mesenchyme containing the common cardinal veins draining into the sinus venosus of the heart. As the two small lung buds grow, they grow into the two pericardioperitoneal canals (which now become the primitive pleural cavity). As the lungs expand and the pleural cavities enlarge, they split the body wall. While the two membranes fuse in the midline, splitting of the body wall continues to form two layers. These two layers are mesenchymal in origin. The outer layer contributes to the thoracic wall and the inner layer (the pleuropericardial membrane) forms the fibrous pericardium enclosing the heart. The inner layer comes to enclose the heart and eventually fuses with the ventral mesentery of the oesophagus. The two lungs are separated from one another by a large mass of mesenchyme lying between the sternum and the vertebral column. This represents the primitive mediastinum.

The right common cardinal vein contributes to the superior vena cava.

The left common cardinal vein forms the oblique vein of the left atrium.

DIVISION OF THE COELOM
61. PLEUROPERICARDIAL MEMBRANES

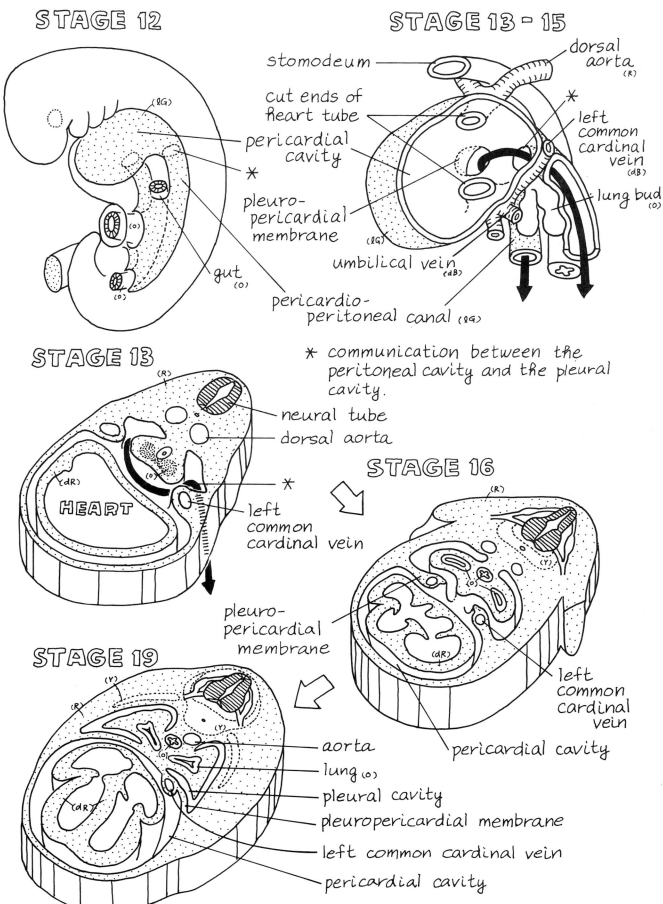

STAGE 12

STAGE 13 - 15

stomodeum

dorsal aorta (R)

cut ends of heart tube

peri cardial cavity

*

left common cardinal vein (dB)

pleuro-pericardial membrane

lung bud (O)

umbilical vein (dB)

pericardio-peritoneal canal (lG)

(lG)

gut (O)

(lG)

(O)

(O)

* communication between the peritoneal cavity and the pleural cavity.

STAGE 13

neural tube

dorsal aorta

(R)

*

(dR)

left common cardinal vein

(O)

HEART

STAGE 16

(R)

pleuro-pericardial membrane

(Y)

(dR)

left common cardinal vein

STAGE 19

(Y)

pericardial cavity

(R)

(Y)

aorta

(O)

lung (O)

pleural cavity

pleuropericardial membrane

left common cardinal vein

(dR)

pericardial cavity

62. Diaphragm (Including Pleuroperitoneal Membranes) Formation

There are four structures which contribute to the formation of the diaphragm: the septum transversum, the pleuroperitoneal membranes, the mesentery of the oesophagus and the body wall.

The septum transversum is composed of mesenchyme and is carried into position during head fold formation (see 12. Head and Tail Folds). It will form the central tendon of the adult diaphragm.

The pleuroperitoneal membranes and pleuropericardial membranes form at approximately the same time. The pleuroperitoneal membranes are caudal partitions which gradually separate from the body wall as the lungs and pleural cavities expand. In Week 6 they extend medially until their free margins fuse with the dorsal mesentery of the oesophagus and septum transversum. As closure occurs, myoblasts (muscle precursor cells) grow into the membranes with their nerve supply from the lower intercostal region. Fusion of these elements closes the pleuroperitoneal canals, and a primitive diaphragm separates the thoracic and abdominal cavities.

Myoblasts also grow into the oesophageal mesentery which forms the median part of the diaphragm. These myoblasts will form the crura of the diaphragm.

During Weeks 9–12, the lungs and pleural cavities split the body wall vertically and produce an inner and outer layer. The inner layer contributes muscle to the diaphragm peripheral to the pleuroperitoneal membranes. The outer layer contributes to the abdominal wall.

As the pleural cavities continue to split the body wall vertically, the costodiaphragmatic recesses are produced and the dome shape of the adult diaphragm is established.

As the various elements of the diaphragm form, their contributions assume different relative importances. Both the septum transversum and pleuroperitoneal membranes comprise large elements in the primitive diaphragm but are small elements in the adult diaphragm. This is particularly true of the pleuroperitoneal membranes.

Anomalies of the Diaphragm

Congenital diaphragmatic hernia may be due to a posterolateral defect in the diaphragm. This often occurs on the left side and results from failure of fusion of the left pleuroperitoneal membrane with the other components of the diaphragm. Herniation of the abdominal viscera into the pleural cavity is often associated with this defect.

62. DIAPHRAGM (INCLUDING PLEURO-PERITONEAL MEMBRANES) FORMATION

STAGE 14

STAGE 17

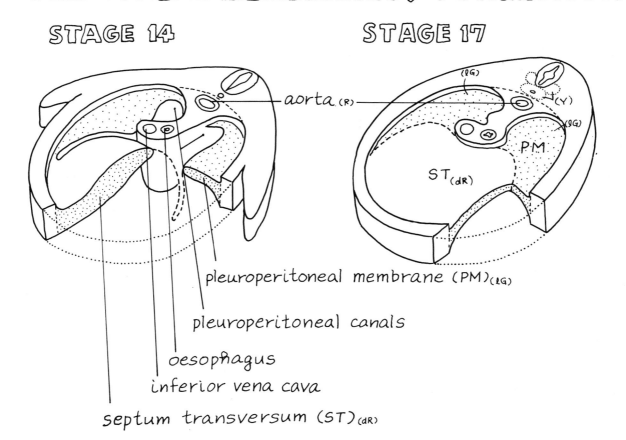

aorta (R)

pleuroperitoneal membrane (PM)(lG)

pleuroperitoneal canals

oesophagus

inferior vena cava

septum transversum (ST)(dR)

WEEK 12

NEW BORN

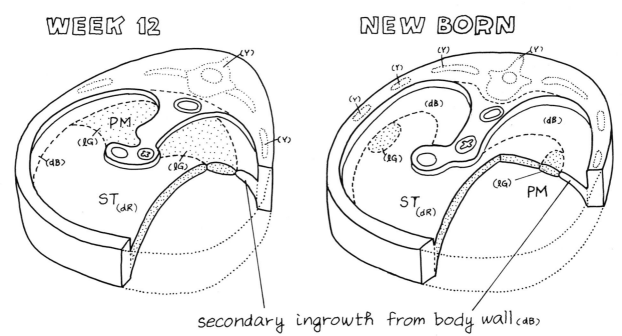

secondary ingrowth from body wall(dB)

63. Positional Changes of the Developing Diaphragm

In Week 4 the septum transversum lies opposite the cervical somites 3, 4, and 5. Developing muscle cells (myoblasts) from these somites migrate into the septum transversum carrying their nerve supply with them from the third, fourth and fifth somites. These nerves will join on each side to form the phrenic nerve.

As the dorsal part of the embryo grows faster than the ventral part, the septum transversum 'migrates' and 'descends' in the body until it reaches the vertebral level, L1. The phrenic nerves lengthen correspondingly as the diaphragm descends in the body.

63. POSITIONAL CHANGES OF THE DEVELOPING DIAPHRAGM

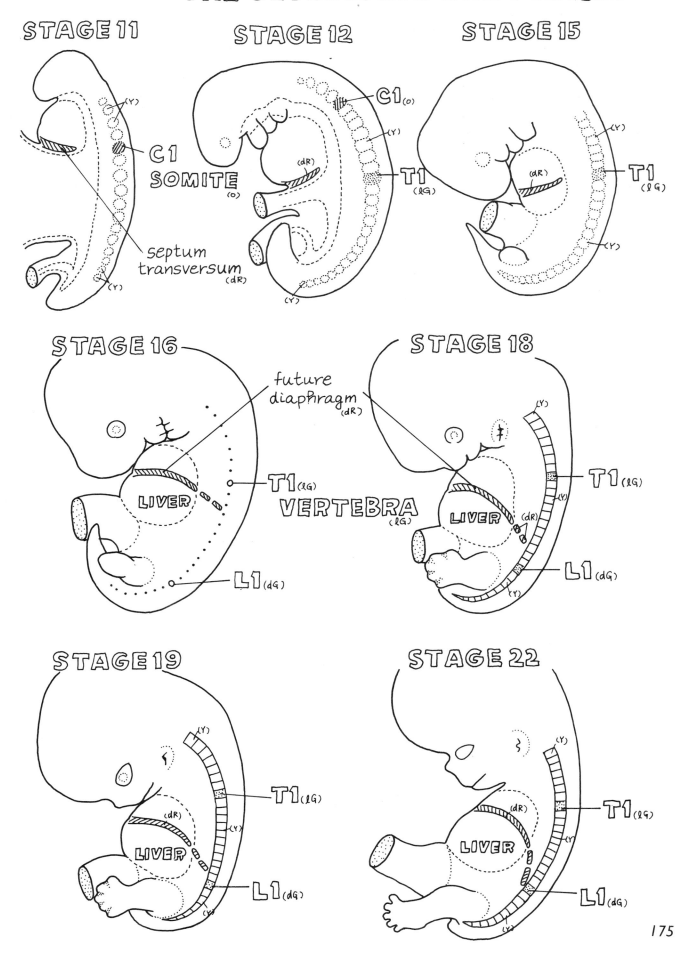

STAGE 11

STAGE 12

STAGE 15

C1 SOMITE

septum transversum

STAGE 16

STAGE 18

future diaphragm

LIVER

VERTEBRA

STAGE 19

STAGE 22

LIVER

LIVER

RESPIRATORY SYSTEM

64. Early Development

In Week 4, the primordium of the lower respiratory system appears as the laryngotracheal groove in the floor of the primitive pharynx (foregut). The groove runs in the midline caudal to the pharyngeal pouches and the hypobranchial eminence. Viewed externally the groove appears as a ridge, called the laryngotracheal diverticulum, and it will give rise to the respiratory system. As the diverticulum grows out into the surrounding splanchnic mesenchyme, it forms a rounded endodermal lung bud which soon re-divides into two bronchial buds. The diverticulum is separated from the foregut (oesophagus) by a partition called the tracheoesophageal septum.

The endodermal laryngotracheal diverticulum will develop into the epithelium of the larynx, trachea, bronchi, bronchioles, pulmonary lining epithelium and secretory epithelial cells of the tracheal glands.

The surrounding splanchnic mesenchyme gives rise to the cartilage, smooth muscle, connective tissue and blood vessels.

RESPIRATORY SYSTEM
64. EARLY DEVELOPMENT
STAGE 12

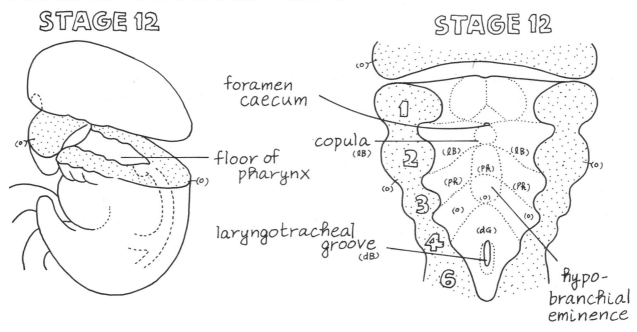

foramen
caecum

floor of
pharynx

copula (ℓB)

laryngotracheal
groove (dB)

STAGE 12

1

2 (ℓB) (ℓB)

(ℓB) (ℓB)

(PR) (PR)

3 (PR) (PR)

(o) (o)

4 (dG)

6

hypo-
branchial
eminence

STAGE 12 - 13

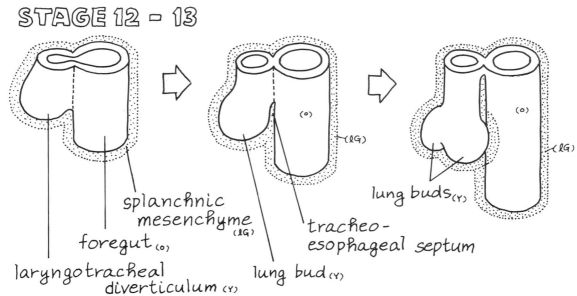

splanchnic
mesenchyme (ℓG)

foregut (o)

laryngotracheal
diverticulum (Y)

lung bud (Y)

tracheo-
esophageal septum

lung buds (Y)

177

65. Larynx

The larynx develops at the cranial end of the laryngotracheal tube. The slit-like inlet from the pharynx forms the laryngeal inlet or aditus. The surrounding splanchnic mesenchyme from the fourth and sixth branchial arches proliferates to form the two arytenoid swellings which grow rostrally towards the tongue. The epiglottis is a derivative of the caudal part of the midline hypobranchial eminence. This eminence is produced by the proliferation of third and fourth branchial arch mesenchyme. As the mesenchyme proliferates, the epiglottal swelling and the two arytenoid swellings convert the laryngeal aditus from a linear to a 'T' shaped entrance.

The remaining laryngeal cartilages (thyroid, cuneiform, cricoid and corniculate) are derivatives of the fourth and sixth branchial arch cartilages. The laryngeal epithelium originates from the endodermal lining of the cranial laryngotracheal tube. It proliferates rapidly and occludes the laryngeal lumen. When recanalisation occurs in Week 10, the laryngeal ventricles, vestibular folds and vocal folds (vocal cords) are apparent. Rarely, incomplete recanalisation results in laryngeal webbing which partly obstructs the airway.

The laryngeal muscles are formed from myoblasts of the fourth and sixth branchial arches. They are supplied by the laryngeal branches of the vagus nerves which supply these arches.

In the newborn, the resting larynx lies at the vertebral level of C2–C3. Later in development, the larynx descends in the neck to levels C3–C4.

65. LARYNX
STAGE 13 - 16

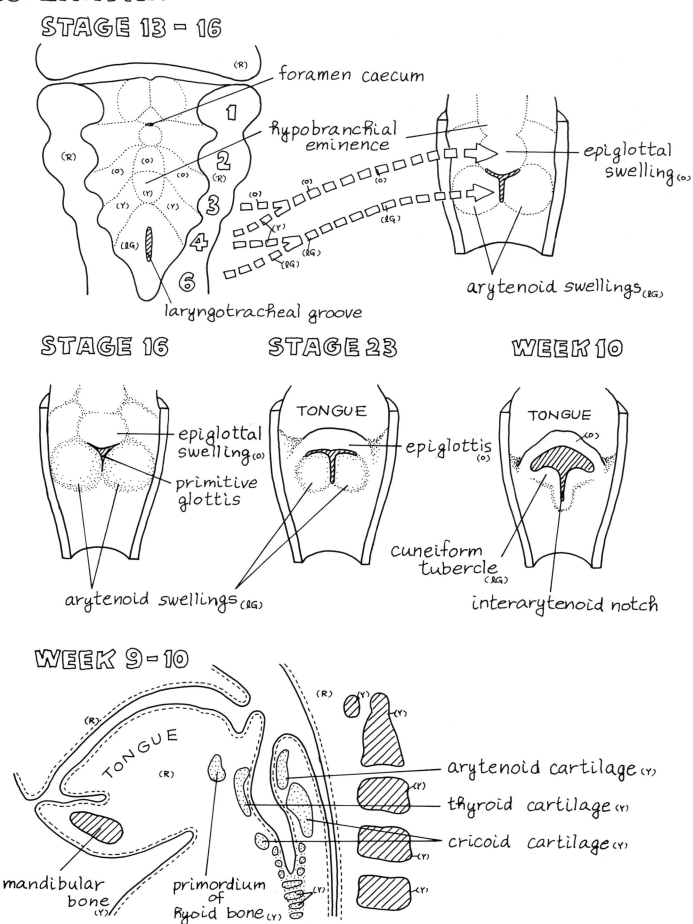

foramen caecum

hypobranchial eminence

(R)

1
2 (R)
3
4
6

(R)

(R) (O) (O) (O)
(O) (Y) (Y)
(O) (LG)

(O) (O) (O)
(Y) (LG)
(Y)
(LG) (LG)
(LG)

epiglottal swelling (O)

arytenoid swellings (LG)

laryngotracheal groove

STAGE 16   STAGE 23   WEEK 10

epiglottal swelling (O)

primitive glottis

arytenoid swellings (LG)

TONGUE

epiglottis (O)

TONGUE

(O)

cuneiform tubercle (LG)

interarytenoid notch

WEEK 9 - 10

(R)

TONGUE

(R) (R)

(R) (Y)

(Y)

(Y) (Y)

(Y)

(Y)

(Y)

arytenoid cartilage (Y)

thyroid cartilage (Y)

cricoid cartilage (Y)

mandibular bone (Y)

primordium of hyoid bone (Y)

66. Trachea

The tracheal epithelium and glands develop from the laryngotracheal tube distal to the larynx. The majority of the glands are present at birth. The surrounding splanchnic mesenchyme forms the muscles, cartilages and connective tissue of the trachea.

The 16–20 tracheal cartilages are present during fetal life. In the newborn, the bifurcation of the trachea is at vertebral levels T3–4, while in the adult it is at T4–5.

Anomalies of the Trachea

A tracheoesophageal fistula is an abnormal canal or communication between the trachea and oesophagus. This is the most common anomaly of the lower respiratory system. It occurs mainly in males and is usually associated with oesophageal atresia. Polyhydramnios (an excess of amniotic fluid) may be associated with these anomalies *in utero.*

66.TRACHEA
STAGE 13

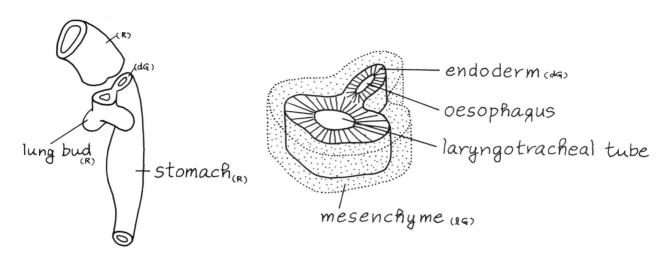

endoderm (dG)

oesophagus

laryngotracheal tube

mesenchyme (lG)

lung bud (R)

stomach (R)

STAGE 16

endoderm (dG)

condensed mesenchyme (lG)

STAGE 18

developing muscle (Y)

epithelium (dG)

developing cartilages (dB)

WEEK 14

muscles (Y)

gland (dG)

cartilage (dB)

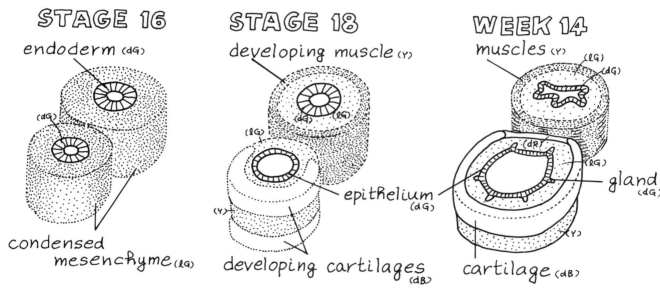

TRACHEOESOPHAGEAL FISTULA
TYPE 1   TYPE 2   TYPE 3   TYPE 4

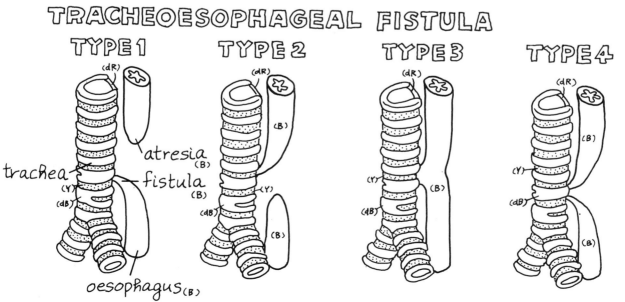

trachea (Y) (dB)

atresia (B)

fistula (B)

oesophagus (B)

67. Bronchi and Lungs

In Week 4, as the single endodermal lung bud grows ventrally into the surrounding splanchnic mesenchyme, it divides into two bronchial buds. Each bud enlarges to form a primary bronchus.

The endodermal buds will form the bronchial system, while the mesenchyme will form the cartilage, smooth muscle, capillaries, connective tissues, and pulmonary connective tissue.

The right primary bronchus is larger and more vertically orientated than the left. The right pulmonary bronchus divides in Week 5 to form two secondary bronchi. The most superior secondary bronchus passes to the superior lobe of the right lung, and the inferior one will re-divide and pass to the middle and inferior lobes. The left lung retains two secondary bronchi supplying the superior and inferior lobes.

During Week 8, the secondary bronchi branch to provide ten segmental (tertiary) bronchi in the right lung and eight or nine in the left lung. Each segmental bronchus with its accompanying mesenchyme forms a bronchopulmonary segment.

As the lungs develop, they grow laterally into the pericardioperitoneal canals which will form the pleural cavities (see **61**. Pleuropericardial Membranes). As they grow, they acquire a visceral pleura from the splanchnic mesenchyme.

Anomalies

Occasionally additional lobes or fissures are present but congenital anomalies of the lungs are uncommon.

67. BRONCHI AND LUNGS

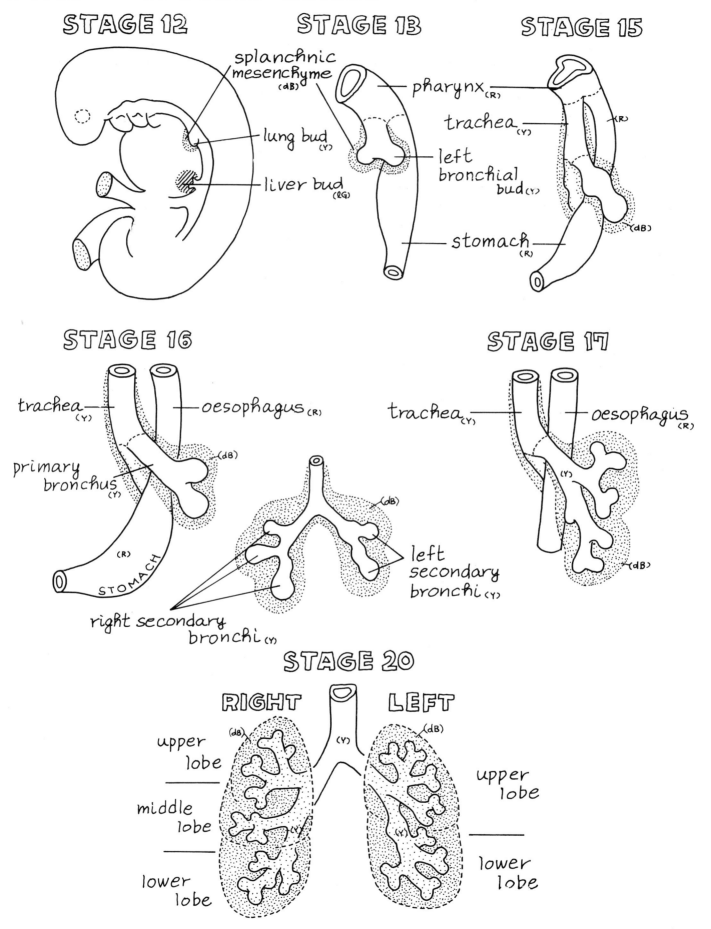

STAGE 12

STAGE 13

splanchnic mesenchyme (dB)

pharynx (R)

lung bud (Y)

liver bud (lG)

trachea (Y)

left bronchial bud (Y)

stomach (R)

STAGE 15

(R)

(dB)

STAGE 16

trachea (Y)

oesophagus (R)

primary bronchus (Y)

(dB)

(R)

STOMACH

right secondary bronchi (Y)

left secondary bronchi (Y)

STAGE 17

trachea (Y)

oesophagus (R)

(Y)

(dB)

STAGE 20

RIGHT

LEFT

(dB)

(Y)

(dB)

upper lobe

upper lobe

middle lobe

(Y)

(Y)

lower lobe

lower lobe

68. Histological Stages of Lung Development

There are four histological stages of lung development which overlap with one another because the cranial segments of the lung mature more rapidly than the caudal segments.

1. *The Pseudoglandular Period (Weeks 5–17)*

   The major elements of the lung have divided only as far as the terminal bronchioles and the lung has a glandular appearance.

2. *The Canalicular Period (Weeks 16–25)*

   The lung tissue becomes highly vascular and the lumina of the bronchi and terminal bronchioles enlarge. Respiratory bronchioles are present, as well as some terminal sacs.

3. *The Terminal Sac Period (Weeks 24–birth)*

   Many terminal sacs develop. Their epithelium thins and capillaries come to lie in close association with them to form primitive alveoli. Two cell types are present: squamous epithelial cells (Type I) and rounded secretory cells (Type II) which secrete surfactant. Surfactant will reduce surface tension and facilitate the expansion of the primitive alveoli during breathing. Thyroxin stimulates the production of surfactant.

4. *The Alveolar Period (late fetal period–8 years of age)*

   The terminal sac epithelium continues to thin and the capillaries bulge into the terminal sacs to form immature alveoli. Until 3 years of age, the lungs grow by the formation of more immature alveoli. From 3–8 years of age, immature alveoli continue to form and to increase in size. Approximately 95% of alveoli develop after birth.

As gaseous exchange cannot occur during the pseudoglandular period, a fetus born in this period cannot survive. Towards the end of the canalicular period, a fetus may survive with intensive care.

Survival of a premature infant is primarily dependent upon the development of the pulmonary vasculature and an adequate supply of surfactant. Both of these things have normally happened to some extent by Weeks 26–28, but the older the infant thereafter the better the chance of survival.

68. HISTOLOGICAL STAGES OF LUNG DEVELOPMENT

WEEK 12

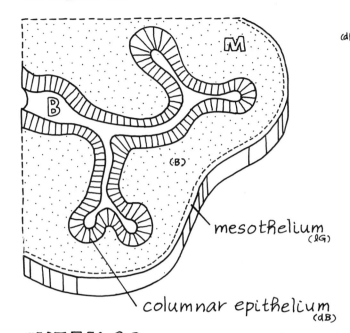

mesothelium (lG)

columnar epithelium (dB)

WEEK 20

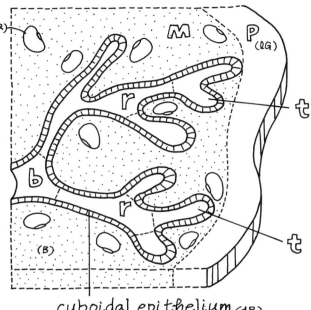

cuboidal epithelium (dB)

WEEK 26

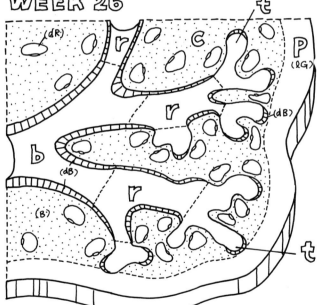

M : MESENCHYME
(future connective tissue)

C : CONNECTIVE TISSUE

P : PLEURA

B : BRONCHUS

b : bronchiole

r : respiratory bronchiole

t : terminal sac

cuboidal epithelium transforming to squamous epithelium

WEEK 26

BRONCHIOLE	RESPIRATORY BRONCHIOLE	FUTURE ALVEOLUS
ciliary epithelium	cuboidal epithelium	squamous epithelium

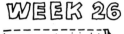

69. Changes at Birth

From Weeks 12–14, fetal breathing movements occur infrequently, but by Week 18 they regularly occur and aspirate amniotic fluid into the lungs. The aspirated fluid mixes with fluid derived from the lungs and tracheal glands.

During birth, most of the fluid is expelled through the mouth and nose as the infant is compressed during its passage down the birth canal. Fluid is also removed via the pulmonary capillaries, and via the lymphatics and pulmonary vessels. A very significant decrease in pulmonary resistance occurs and allows a marked increase in blood flow from the pulmonary trunk.

Respiratory distress syndrome in the neonate is characterised by rapid, laboured breathing. A major cause of this syndrome is hyaline membrane disease in which there is a deficiency of surfactant. The lungs are underinflated and have a characteristic glossy, hyaline membrane.

69. CHANGES AT BIRTH

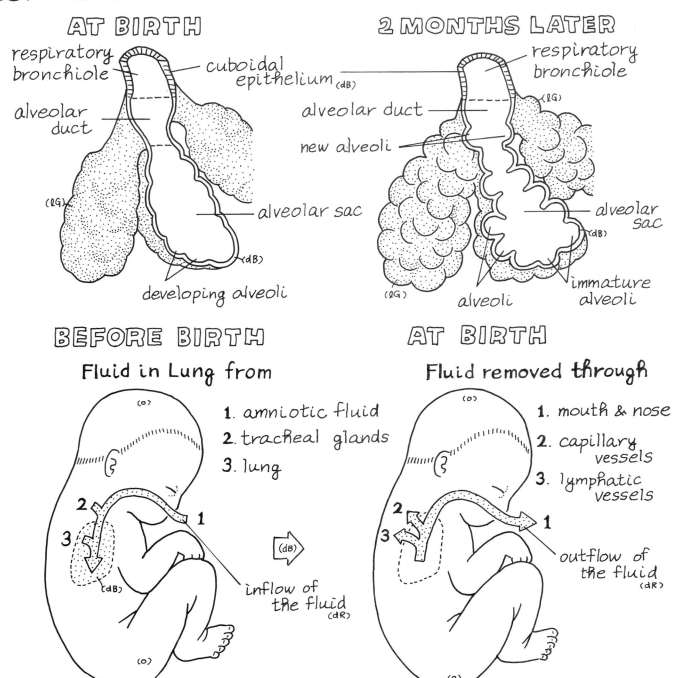

AT BIRTH

respiratory bronchiole

cuboidal epithelium (dB)

alveolar duct

(lG)

alveolar sac

(dB)

developing alveoli

2 MONTHS LATER

respiratory bronchiole

(lG)

alveolar duct

new alveoli

alveolar sac

(dB)

(lG)

alveoli

immature alveoli

BEFORE BIRTH

Fluid in Lung from

(o)

2

3

(dB)

(o)

1. amniotic fluid
2. tracheal glands
3. lung

(dB)

inflow of the fluid (dR)

AT BIRTH

Fluid removed through

(o)

2

3

1

(o)

1. mouth & nose
2. capillary vessels
3. lymphatic vessels

outflow of the fluid (dR)

DIGESTIVE SYSTEM

70. Early Gut

In Week 4, the head, tail and lateral body folds incorporate part of the yolk sac adjacent to the embryonic axis. The primitive gut which is incorporated in the region of the head fold becomes the foregut; that in the tail fold becomes the hindgut and that in the middle, which is still in direct communication with the yolk sac, becomes the midgut. However, the embryonic foregut, midgut and hindgut do not correspond exactly to the same regions in the adult. The primitive gut is endoderm-lined and will give rise to the majority of the epithelium and associated parenchyma of the glands of the digestive tract. Surrounding splanchnic mesenchyme will develop into most of the muscles and other tissues of the digestive tract.

As the embryo grows, more and more of the yolk sac is incorporated and the foregut and hindgut lengthen at the expense of the midgut. By Week 20, the very narrow yolk stalk is connected to a small yolk sac which is by then incorporated into the placenta.

The foregut derivatives are:

1. Pharynx and its derivatives
2. Lower respiratory tract
3. Oesophagus
4. Stomach
5. Liver
6. Pancreas
7. Gall bladder
8. Biliary duct system
9. Duodenum cephalic to the opening of the bile duct

The midgut derivatives are:

1. Small intestine including the duodenum distal to the opening of the bile duct
2. Caecum
3. Vermiform appendix
4. Ascending colon
5. Proximal two-thirds of transverse colon

The hindgut derivatives are:

1. Distal one-third of transverse colon
2. Descending colon
3. Sigmoid colon
4. Rectum
5. Superior part of anal canal
6. Epithelium of urinary bladder and most of urethra

The majority of the foregut is supplied by the coeliac artery, the midgut by the superior mesenteric artery, and the hindgut by the inferior mesenteric artery.

DIGESTIVE SYSTEM

70. EARLY GUT
STAGE 9

oropharyngeal
membrane

cloacal membrane

chorionic
villi

(LG)

(O)

allantoic
diverticulum

STAGE 10

(dB)

(dR)

hindgut

(Y)

midgut

(O)

(O)

foregut

allantois

STAGE 11

(dR)

(dB)

midgut

(Y)

(O)

(O)

oropharyngeal membrane

cloacal
membrane

STAGE 12

(dB)

(dR)

foregut

midgut

(Y)

hindgut

(O)

THE DERIVATIVES OF PRIMITIVE GUT

F foregut derivatives

M midgut derivatives

H hindgut derivatives

1 (dB)

2 (dB)

3 (dB)

LUNG
(dB)

5
(dB)

8
(dB)

4

7
(dB)

9
(dB)

6 (dB)

F

M

H

(dR)

5 (dR)

4
(dR)

1

0 1 (Y)

2

(Y)

2
(dR)

(dR)

3 (dR)

3
(Y)

6
(Y)

4
(Y)

5 (Y)

71. Foregut: Oesophagus

The oesophagus is a derivative of the foregut. The tracheoesophageal septum in Week 4 separates it from the laryngotracheal tube. The oesophageal epithelium and its associated glands are endodermal derivatives, whilst mesenchyme surrounding the oesophagus will condense to form the muscles. The muscles of the upper third are striated and originate from the mesenchyme of the caudal branchial arches. The muscles of the middle third are a mixture of striated and smooth muscles, whilst those of the lower third are primarily smooth muscle derived from the surrounding splanchnic mesenchyme. The vagus nerves derived from Branchial Arches IV and VI, supply the striated muscle while a visceral plexus derived from the neural crest cells supplies the smooth muscle.

The oesophagus rapidly lengthens with the relative growth of the embryo and the associated descent of the heart.

The early oesophagus is lined by a simple columnar epithelium. This grows rapidly and fills the lumen of the oesophagus. Functionally, the lumen is almost obliterated until it recanalises (Week 8). Once the lumen is re-established, the epithelium is a pseudostratified ciliated columnar epithelium.

By Week 14 the epithelium is largely changing to the stratified squamous type found in the newborn. In the adult, areas denuded of stratified squamous epithelium due to oesophageal reflux are replaced by columnar epithelium. This is called Barrat's oesophagus.

Anomalies

Oesophageal anomalies found in the fetus include stenosis and atresia; these often are a result of incomplete recanalisation. Incomplete separation of the oesophagus and laryngotracheal tube by the tracheoesophageal septum may result in a tracheoesophageal fistula and atresia of the oesophagus.

71. FOREGUT: OESOPHAGUS

STAGE 13 STAGE 15

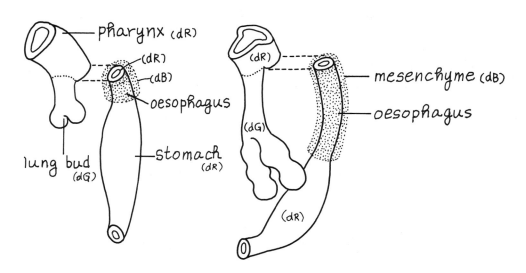

pharynx (dR)

(dR)

(dB)

oesophagus

lung bud (dG)

stomach (dR)

mesenchyme (dB)

oesophagus

(dR)

(dG)

(dR)

0

STAGE 13-14 STAGE 18-19 STAGE 22-23

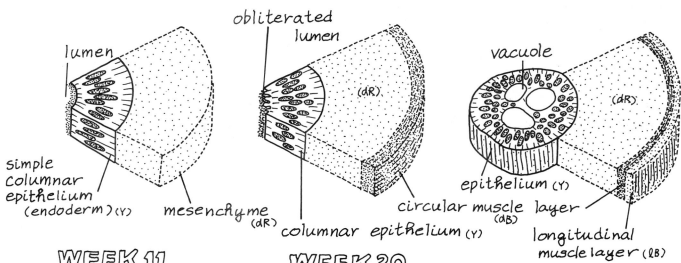

lumen

simple columnar epithelium (endoderm) (Y)

mesenchyme (dR)

obliterated lumen

(dR)

columnar epithelium (Y)

vacuole

(dR)

epithelium (Y)

circular muscle layer (dB)

longitudinal muscle layer (ℓB)

WEEK 11 WEEK 30

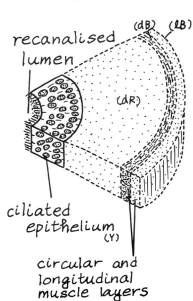

recanalised lumen

(dB) (ℓB)

(dR)

ciliated epithelium (Y)

circular and longitudinal muscle layers

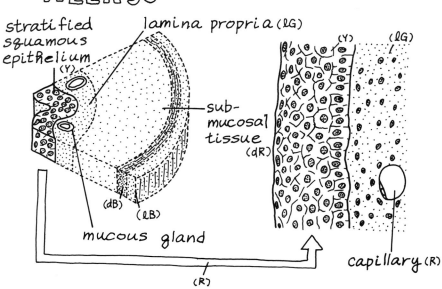

stratified squamous epithelium (Y)

lamina propria (ℓG)

sub-mucosal tissue (dR)

(dB)

(ℓB)

mucous gland

(R)

(Y) (ℓG)

capillary (R)

72. Foregut: Stomach and Greater Omentum

The stomach is a derivative of the foregut and initially it is a straight tube. In Week 4 a dilatation marks the site of the stomach. With further development, the dorsal border grows more rapidly than the ventral border and establishes the greater curvature of the stomach. The ventral border becomes the lesser curvature and the stomach assumes its characteristic 'J' shape. The right and left sides of the stomach are innervated by the right and left vagus nerves. Rennin has been identified in gastric secretions by Week 18.

Rotation

The 'J' shaped stomach slowly rotates, so that the lesser curvature faces the right side of the body and the greater curvature the left side. As this rotation occurs, the stomach also tilts 90° clockwise so its long axis comes to lie almost transverse to the longitudinal body axis. This is why the right vagus nerve in the adult lies on the dorsal surface and the left vagus nerve on the ventral surface. This rotation is directly related to midgut rotation (see **78**. Midgut: Rotation).

Mesenteries

In the early embryo (Week 4), the stomach is suspended from the dorsal body wall by the dorsal mesentery (dorsal mesogastrium). The stomach is also attached (with the cranial part of the duodenum) to the ventral wall by the ventral mesentery (ventral mesogastrium).

The cavity of the entire abdomen is referred to as the greater sac of the peritoneum. There is also a lesser sac of the peritoneum (omental bursa). The omental bursa is closely associated with the dorsal mesogastrium. The dorsal and ventral mesenteries are mesenchymal in origin. The dorsal mesogastrium initially is a thick mesentery, but with development, spaces appear between the cells on the right aspect of the dorsal mesogastrium. These spaces enlarge and then coalesce to form a larger space, the primordium of the omental bursa. As the stomach rotates, the dorsal mesogastrium (and omental bursa) which is attached to the greater curvature, is carried to the left side of the body. Here it hangs off the greater curvature like a large sac. The sac will form the greater omentum of the adult, while the space within is the omental bursa or lesser sac of the peritoneum. The lesser sac communicates with the greater sac of peritoneum via a narrow opening called the epiploic foramen (foramen of Winslow).

The superior part of the lesser sac is cut off as the diaphragm develops. This extension has a superior half, the infracardiac bursa, which normally disappears and an inferior half which persists to form the superior recess of the lesser sac. The inferior recess of the lesser sac exists between the layers of the greater omentum but almost disappears as the layers of the omentum fuse later in development.

Stomach Anomalies

The most common anomaly is congenital pyloric stenosis.

72. FOREGUT: STOMACH AND GREATER OMENTUM

STAGE 13

stomach (Y)

liver bud

STAGE 13 - 18

dorsal mesentery (ℓG)

(ℓG) (Y)

(Y) (dR)

(Y)

(Y) (dR)

(ℓG) (dR)

(dR)

(ℓG) (Y)

ventral mesentery (dR)

STAGE 13

dorsal mesentery (ℓG)

(ℓG) (Y)

(Y)

superior recess (Y)

(ℓG) (Y)

(dR) (Y)

(ℓG)

STAGE 15 - 16

(ℓG) (Y)

infra-cardiac bursa

(ℓG)

(dR) (Y)

(Y)

(ℓG)

(dR) (Y)

spleen (dR)

(Y)

epiploic foramen

STAGE 17 - 18

(ℓG) (Y)

infra-cardiac bursa

(ℓG) (Y)

(ℓG)

(dR) (Y)

(Y)

(ℓG)

(dR) (Y)

(Y)

(ventral mesentery removed)

STAGE 19

(ℓG) (Y)

(Y)

(ℓG)

(ℓG)

(dR) (Y)

spleen (dR)

(ℓG)

(ℓG) (Y)

lesser sac

(dR) (Y)

(ℓG) (Y)

greater omentum

(Y)

(ℓG)

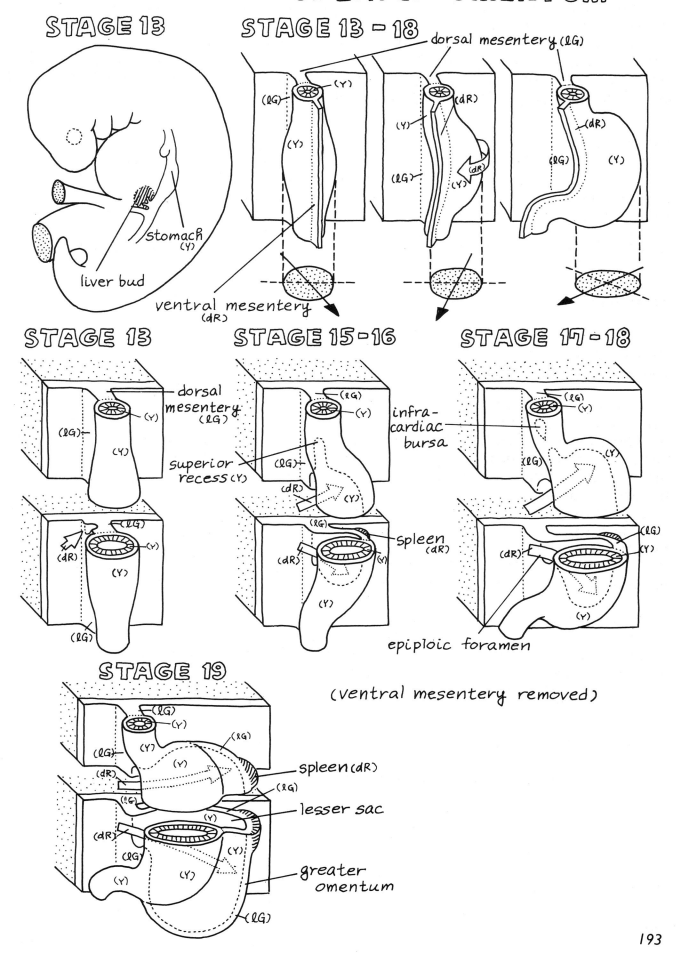

73. Foregut: Liver

Early in Week 4, a ventral endodermal bud arising from the caudal foregut forms the hepatic diverticulum. This will give rise to the liver, gall bladder and biliary duct system. As the endodermal bud grows, cords of cells extend into the mesenchymal mass of the septum transversum and the bud soon divides into two. The most cranial of these two buds will form the parenchyma of the liver; whilst the most caudal forms the gall bladder and cystic duct. The parenchyma of the adult liver is derived from the hepatic diverticulum, while its Kupffer cells, haemopoietic cells, blood vessels and connective tissue arise from the septum transversum.

The liver initially has right and left main lobes of approximately equal size. With development, the right lobe grows faster than the left and the characteristic adult shape is acquired. The quadrate lobe and part of the caudate lobe are derivatives of the right main lobe, but are functionally part of the left main lobe due to their blood supply.

The liver functions as an haemopoietic centre, beginning in Week 6, peaking between the third and sixth months and ceasing by birth.

Bile is formed from Week 12, and by Week 13, it colours the intestinal contents (meconium) dark green.

Ventral Mesentery

The hepatic diverticulum is a ventral outgrowth of the foregut and grows between the two layers of the ventral mesentery. The adult derivatives of the ventral mesentery are:
1. The lesser omentum extending from the liver to the lesser curvature of the stomach (hepatogastric ligament) and from the liver to the duodenum (hepatoduodenal ligament).
2. The falciform ligament (containing the umbilical vein) extending from the liver to the ventral abdominal wall.
3. The visceral peritoneum of the liver.

Ductus Venosus

Blood entering the fetus through the umbilical vein travels to the inferior vena cava via one of two routes. Approximately half enters the hepatic sinusoids and the remainder goes through the ductus venosus and bypasses the liver.

More blood can be made to enter the liver substance when the physiological sphincter of the umbilical vein contracts; this forces the blood into the portal sinus and thence to the portal vein and sinusoids. When the sphincter relaxes, blood flows directly into the ductus venosus and into the inferior vena cava bypassing the liver (see **31**. Changes at Birth).

Anomalies of the Liver

Severe anomalies of the liver are rare, but minor variations occur in lobulation and in the hepatic ducts.

73. FOREGUT: LIVER

STAGE 13

STAGE 13

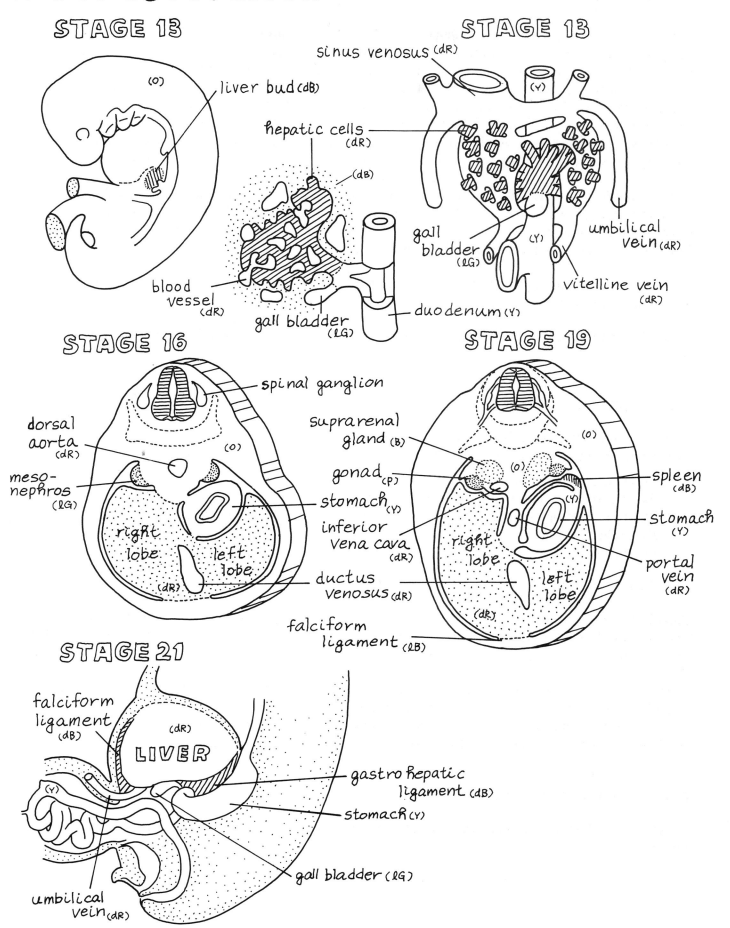

liver bud (dB)

hepatic cells (dR)

(dB)

blood vessel (dR)

gall bladder (lG)

duodenum (Y)

sinus venosus (dR)

(Y)

gall bladder (lG)

umbilical vein (dR)

vitelline vein (dR)

STAGE 16

STAGE 19

dorsal aorta (dR)

meso-nephros (lG)

spinal ganglion

suprarenal gland (B)

gonad (P)

stomach (Y)

inferior vena cava (dR)

ductus venosus (dR)

spleen (dB)

stomach (Y)

portal vein (dR)

right lobe

left lobe

(dR)

right lobe

left lobe

(dR)

(O)

(O)

(Y)

falciform ligament (lB)

STAGE 21

falciform ligament (dB)

(dR)

LIVER

(Y)

gastrohepatic ligament (dB)

stomach (Y)

gall bladder (lG)

umbilical vein (dR)

74. Foregut: Gall Bladder

The gall bladder develops in Week 4 as a solid endodermal outgrowth of the caudal part of the hepatic diverticulum. The stalk of the gall bladder will form the adult cystic duct, while the stalk connecting the hepatic and cystic ducts to the duodenum will form the adult bile duct. By Week 7, vacuoles and degeneration appear in the solid extrabiliary apparatus and later in Week 7, the apparatus is canalised.

When the duodenum rotates during Weeks 5–7, the entrance of the bile duct, which was initially on the ventral surface of the duodenum, is carried around to the dorsal aspect.

By Week 13, bile pigment is secreted which colours the intestinal contents (meconium) dark green. Meconium is not normally present in the amniotic fluid and when found may be indicative of fetal distress due to hypoxia.

Anomalies of the Extrabiliary Apparatus

Failure of the extrabiliary apparatus to canalise in Week 7 results in atresia and the neonate becomes jaundiced because bilirubin is no longer excreted across the placenta.

74. FOREGUT: GALL BLADDER

STAGE 13

STAGE 13

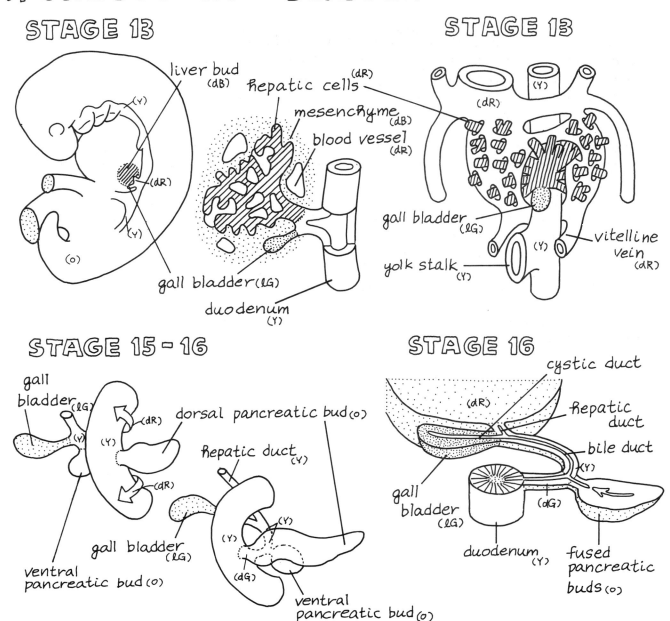

liver bud (dB)

hepatic cells (dR)

mesenchyme (dB)

blood vessel (dR)

(Y)

(dR)

(dR)

(Y)

(o)

gall bladder (lG)

duodenum (Y)

gall bladder (lG)

yolk stalk (Y)

vitelline vein (dR)

(Y)

STAGE 15-16

STAGE 16

gall bladder (lG)

(dR)

(Y)

(Y)

dorsal pancreatic bud (o)

hepatic duct (Y)

gall bladder (lG)

ventral pancreatic bud (o)

(Y)

(Y)

(dG)

ventral pancreatic bud (o)

cystic duct

hepatic duct

bile duct (Y)

(dR)

gall bladder (lG)

duodenum (Y)

(dG)

fused pancreatic buds (o)

75. Foregut: Pancreas

The pancreas develops in Week 5 from dorsal and ventral endodermal buds arising from the caudal foregut; these give rise to the parenchyma of the gland. The septa and connective tissue capsule arise from adjacent splanchnic mesenchyme.

The dorsal pancreatic bud is larger and lies on the dorsal aspect of the foregut. Its origin is cephalic to that of the smaller ventral pancreatic bud which lies on the ventral aspect near the entrance of the bile duct into the duodenum. Each bud has a duct system. The dorsal bud grows into the dorsal mesentery and forms most of the pancreas: part of the head of the pancreas, the body and tail of the adult pancreas.

During rotation of the stomach and midgut rotation, the ventral pancreatic bud and its duct are carried dorsally (clockwise) where they fuse with the dorsal pancreatic bud and its duct system. The ventral pancreatic bud will form the uncinate process and part of the head of the adult pancreas.

The main pancreatic duct of the adult forms from the duct of the ventral bud and the distal portion of the dorsal bud duct. The proximal portion of the dorsal bud duct may persist as an accessory pancreatic duct.

Insulin and glucagon are present by Week 20.

Anomalies of the Pancreas

Anomalies of the pancreas include accessory pancreatic tissue, often located heterotypically in the wall of the stomach, duodenum, or in Meckel's diverticulum.

The rarer anular pancreas is a ring of pancreatic tissue which forms around the duodenum. It is believed to form when a bifid ventral pancreatic bud grows around the duodenum and fuses with the dorsal bud. This may cause duodenal obstruction in the neonate.

75. FOREGUT: PANCREAS

STAGE 13

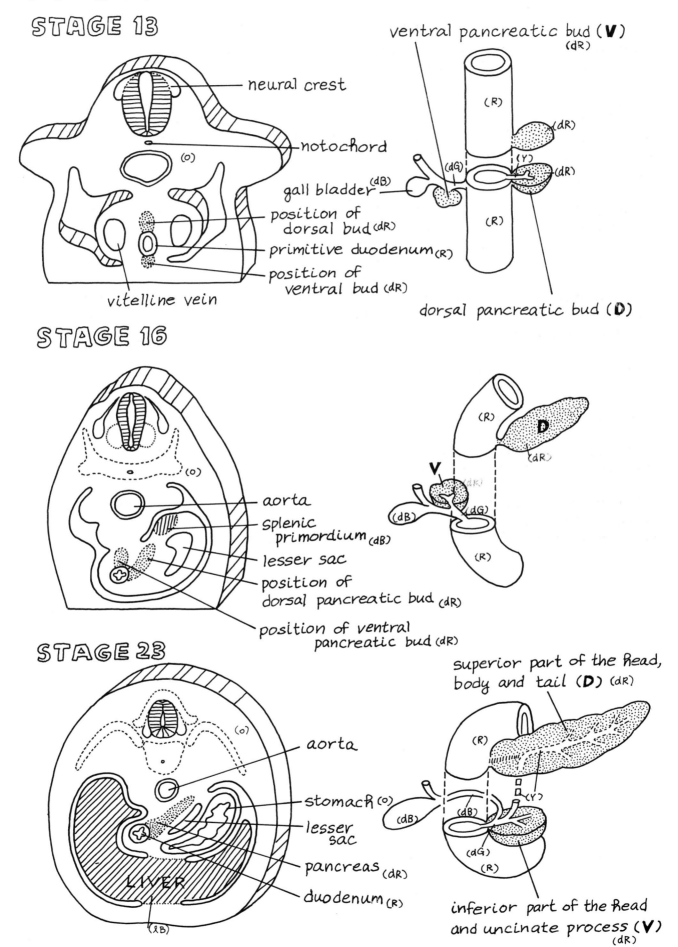

neural crest

notochord

(O)

gall bladder (dB)

position of dorsal bud (dR)

primitive duodenum (R)

position of ventral bud (dR)

vitelline vein

ventral pancreatic bud (**V**) (dR)

(R)

(dR)

(dG)   (Y)

(dR)

(R)

dorsal pancreatic bud (**D**)

STAGE 16

(O)

aorta

Splenic primordium (dB)

lesser sac

position of dorsal pancreatic bud (dR)

position of ventral pancreatic bud (dR)

(R)

D

(dR)

V

(dR)

(dB)

(dG)

(R)

STAGE 23

(O)

aorta

stomach (O)

lesser sac

pancreas (dR)

duodenum (R)

LIVER

(lB)

superior part of the head, body and tail (**D**) (dR)

(R)

(Y)

(dB)   (dB)

(dG)

(R)

inferior part of the head and uncinate process (**V**) (dR)

76. Foregut and Midgut: Duodenum

The duodenum has a dual origin from the endoderm of the caudal foregut and the cephalic midgut. The muscles form from the surrounding splanchnic mesenchyme.

In Week 4, the duodenum begins to develop and grows rapidly to produce a 'C' shaped loop directed ventrally. In the embryo, the apex of the duodenal loop represents the junction between the parts derived from foregut and midgut. This junction in the adult is just distal to the entrance of the bile duct. The region originating from the foregut is supplied by branches of the coeliac artery, while that from the midgut by the superior mesenteric artery.

The position of the duodenum is affected during rotation of the stomach and midgut. The 'C' shaped loop is carried to the right where it is pressed against the posterior abdominal wall by the colon. Adjacent layers of peritoneum fuse and disappear so that most of the duodenum becomes retroperitoneal (behind the peritoneum).

STAGE 13

STAGE 13

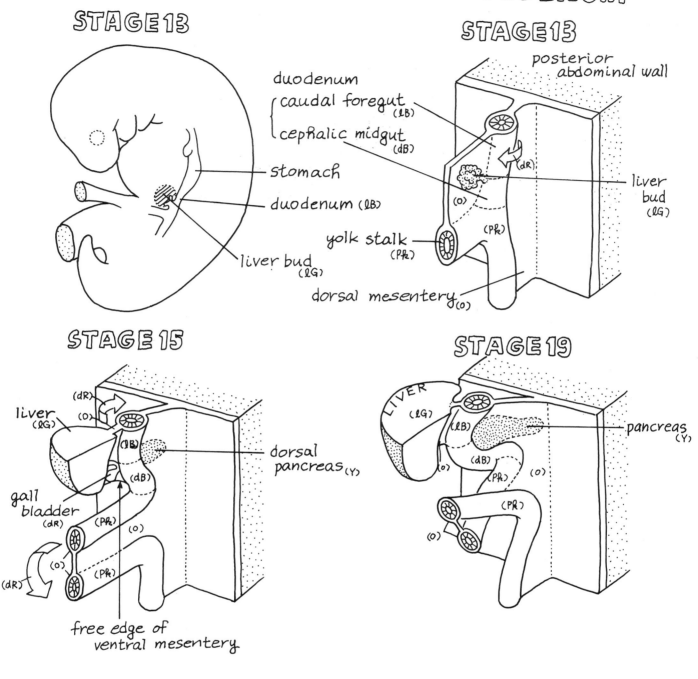

duodenum

caudal foregut (ℓB)

cephalic midgut (dB)

stomach

duodenum (ℓB)

liver bud (ℓG)

posterior abdominal wall

(dR)

liver bud (ℓG)

yolk stalk (Pℛ)

(o)

dorsal mesentery (o)

STAGE 15

liver (ℓG)

(dR)

(o)

(ℓB)

(dB)

gall bladder (dR)

(Pℛ)

(o)

(o)

(Pℛ)

(dR)

dorsal pancreas (Y)

free edge of ventral mesentery

STAGE 19

LIVER (ℓG)

(ℓB)

(dB)

(Pℛ)

(o)

(o)

(Pℛ)

pancreas (Y)

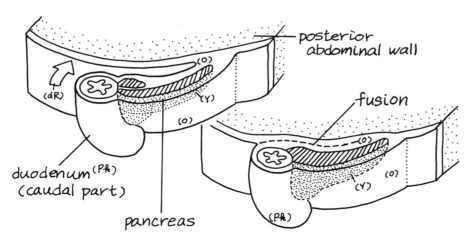

posterior abdominal wall

(o)

(dR)

(Y)

(o)

fusion

(o)

duodenum (Pℛ) (caudal part)

pancreas

(Y)

(Pℛ)

In Weeks 5–6, the epithelium proliferates rapidly and fills the lumen which is almost functionally obliterated until Week 8 when it becomes recanalised. Brunner's glands appear in the third month.

Anomalies of the Duodenum

The most frequently occurring anomaly is duodenal stenosis. This may be due to failure of recanalisation or the result of an anular pancreas.

Duodenal atresia is not common but when present is often associated with other severe congenital anomalies.

STAGE 13

STAGE 16

STAGE 17-19

STAGE 22

endodermal
epithelium
(ℓG)

mesenchyme
(ℓB)

obliterated
lumen

(ℓG)

(ℓB)

developing circular
muscle layer (dB)

(ℓG)

(ℓB)

(dB)

vacuole

primitive
villi (ℓB)

columnar
epithelium
(ℓG)

(ℓB)

inner circular
muscle layer (dB)

77. Spleen

In Week 5, the spleen begins to form from islands of mesenchymal cells between the layers of the dorsal mesogastrium. These islands coalesce and the resulting fetal spleen is lobulated. Late in fetal life, the lobules fuse and the only remnants of the lobulation are notches along the superior border.

The mesenchymal cells form the capsule, parenchyma and connective tissue of the spleen. The haemopoietic cells are currently believed to arise *de novo* rather than to have originated from the yolk sac. Until late fetal life, the spleen is an haemopoietic organ but in the neonate and adult, blood cells are not normally produced by the spleen.

Anomalies of the Spleen

The most common anomalies are accessory spleens which are found near the hilum of the spleen, in the tail of the pancreas, or in the gastrolienal ligament.

77. SPLEEN

STAGE 13

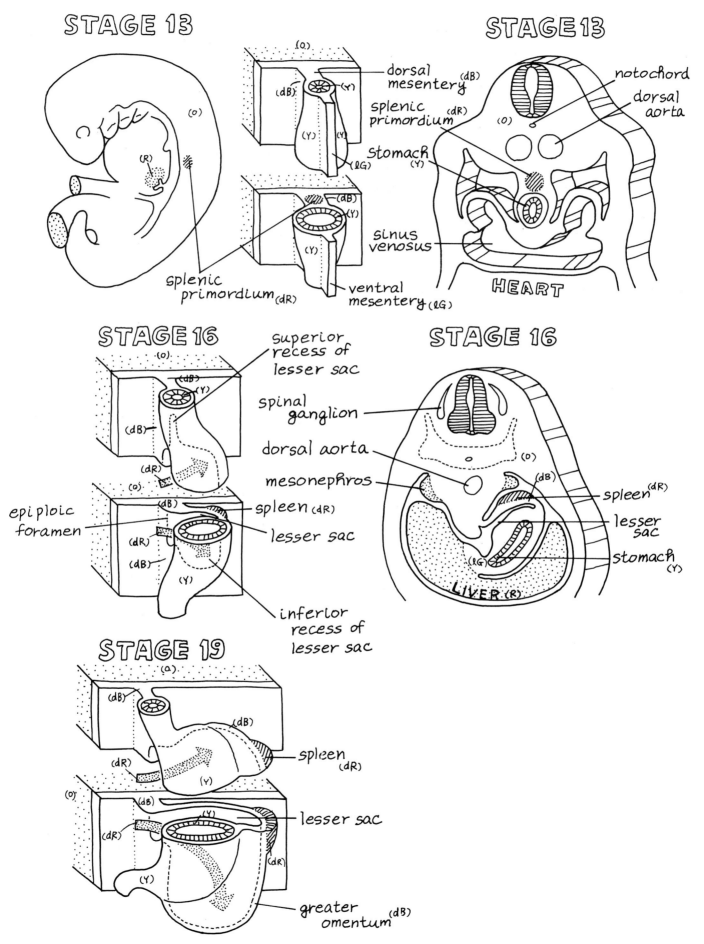

dorsal mesentery (dB)

splenic primordium (dR)

Stomach (Y)

splenic primordium (dR)

ventral mesentery (lG)

STAGE 13

notochord

dorsal aorta

sinus venosus

HEART

STAGE 16

superior recess of lesser sac

spinal ganglion

dorsal aorta

mesonephros

epiploic foramen

spleen (dR)

lesser sac

inferior recess of lesser sac

STAGE 16

spleen (dR)

lesser sac

stomach (Y)

LIVER (R)

STAGE 19

spleen (dR)

lesser sac

greater omentum (dB)

78. Midgut: Rotation

During Week 6, the midgut rapidly elongates and herniates into the extraembryonic coelom within the umbilical cord. In this position, the midgut loop will undergo rotation before re-entering the abdominal cavity (Week 10) to assume its definitive position. As the midgut returns to the abdominal cavity, the connection between the extraembryonic and intraembryonic coelom via the umbilicus is obliterated. The different regions become distinct later in development (Week 18).

There are two easily identifiable landmarks on the midgut loop which may be used to understand the process of rotation. Firstly, at the midpoint of the loop, the remnant of the yolk stalk (vitello-intestinal duct) demarcates the cranial (proximal) segment and the caudal (distal) segment of the loop. Secondly, the caecal diverticulum on the caudal segment marks the future site of the caecum and vermiform appendix. The midgut is supplied by the superior mesenteric artery and is suspended from the dorsal aspect of the abdominal wall by the dorsal mesentery.

Rotation occurs in five major, continuous steps. If the observer faces the ventral aspect of the embryo, all rotation is in an anticlockwise direction.

1. The midgut loop rotates 90° anticlockwise and comes to lie in the horizontal plane. The cranial segment is on the embryo's right and the caudal segment on the left.
2. The cranial segment increases greatly in length to form the coils of the jejunum and ileum.
3. The cranial segment (jejunum and ileum) returns to the abdominal cavity. As it returns, it undergoes further anticlockwise rotation and passes posterior to the superior mesenteric artery into the centre and then moves to the left, posterior side of the abdominal cavity.
4. As the caudal midgut segment now returns to the abdominal cavity, it rotates further in an anticlockwise direction. The transverse colon comes to lie cephalic to the superior mesenteric artery and the caecum on the right side of the abdominal cavity.
5. The caecum gradually descends to the right iliac fossa by differential growth. The parts of the colon are now distinct: i.e., ascending, transverse and descending segments.

Midgut Anomalies

There are various congenital abnormalities of the intestines:

Reverse rotation
The transverse colon crosses posterior to the superior mesenteric artery and the duodenum anterior to the artery.

Non-rotation
The small intestine comes to lie on the right side, and the large intestine on the left.

Non-return of herniated midgut
Omphalocoele: loops of intestine remain herniated in a sac of peritoneum and amnion.

Umbilical hernia
The abdominal contents herniate after their return through an imperfectly closed linea alba. The hernia is covered by skin and subcutaneous tissue.

Meckel's diverticulum
Persistent yolk stalk.

Incomplete descent of the caecum
Sub-hepatic: i.e., below the liver.

Stenosis (narrowing) and atresia (complete obstruction)
May result from incomplete or failure of recanalisation. This occurs most often in the duodenum and ileum.

78. MIDGUT: ROTATION

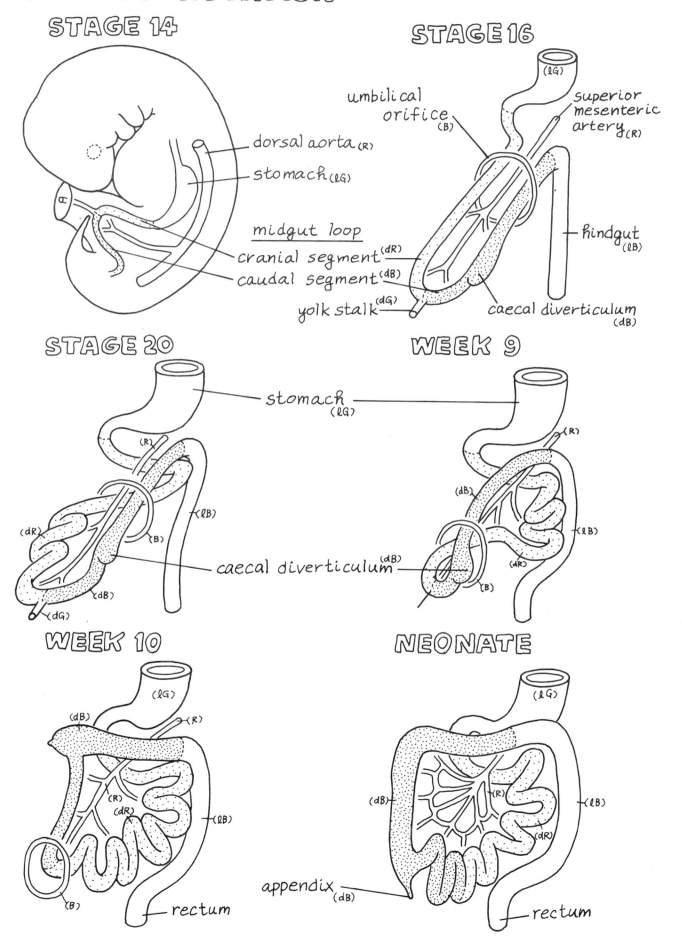

STAGE 14

dorsal aorta (R)

stomach (ℓG)

midgut loop
cranial segment (dR)

caudal segment (dB)

STAGE 16

(ℓG)

umbilical orifice (B)

superior mesenteric artery (R)

hindgut (ℓB)

yolk stalk (dG)

caecal diverticulum (dB)

STAGE 20

stomach (ℓG)

(R)

(dR)

(B)

(ℓB)

caecal diverticulum (dB)

(dB)

(dG)

WEEK 9

(R)

(dB)

(ℓB)

caecal diverticulum (dB)

(dR)

(B)

WEEK 10

(ℓG)

(dB)

(R)

(R)

(dR)

(ℓB)

(B)

rectum

NEONATE

(ℓG)

(dB)

(R)

(ℓB)

(dR)

appendix (dB)

rectum

79. Fixation of Intestines

Before the midgut rotates, all parts have a mesentery suspending them from the posterior abdominal wall. During rotation, parts of the mesentery become twisted around the superior mesenteric artery. After rotation, some of the mesenteries will fuse with the parietal peritoneum of the posterior abdominal wall and become 'fixed'. This happens to the mesentery of most of the duodenum and the mesenteries of the ascending colon and descending colon and these three parts of the gut become retroperitoneal. The remaining mesentery does not fuse with the posterior abdominal wall so that the small intestine, transverse mesocolon and sigmoid colon remain mobile within the abdominal cavity.

Errors of Fixation

Parts of the intestine which are normally retroperitoneal have a mesentery and are more mobile. These may twist (volvulus) and obstruct their own blood supply.

Parts of the intestine which normally have a mesentery may lack one and be fixed.

79. FIXATION OF INTESTINES

MESENTERY BEFORE FIXATION

MESENTERY FIXED IN SHADED AREA

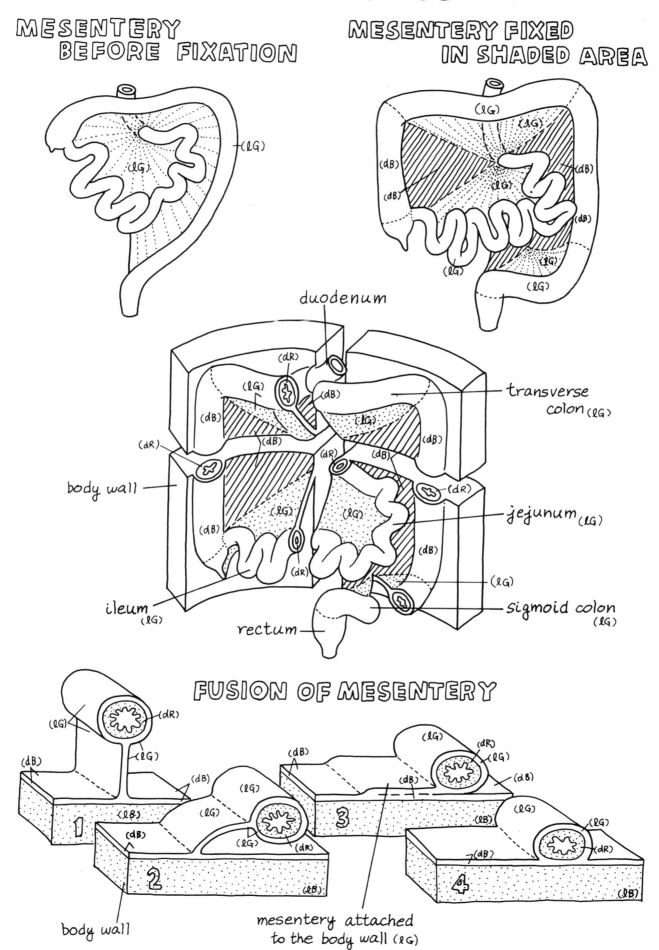

duodenum

transverse colon (lG)

body wall

jejunum (lG)

(dR)

ileum (lG)

rectum

sigmoid colon (lG)

FUSION OF MESENTERY

body wall

mesentery attached to the body wall (lG)

80. Caecum and Vermiform Appendix

In Week 6, the caecal diverticulum forms on the caudal limb of the midgut loop. This develops into the caecum and appendix. The most cephalic part of the diverticulum, which will form the caecum, grows more rapidly than the caudal part of the diverticulum, which will form the appendix. As a result, the appendix is identifiable in Week 7, and becomes a relatively long, finger-like tube by birth. It projects in a direction continuous with the midline of the caecum. After birth, it changes its position due to differential growth of the caecum.

The position of the embryonic caecal diverticulum is a constant and useful marker to follow during midgut rotation (see **78**. Midgut: Rotation). Only after birth does the appendix become very variable in position. The most frequent position (64% of adults) is retrocaecal (behind the caecum).

80. CAECUM AND VERMIFORM APPENDIX

STAGE 16 STAGE 21 WEEK 11

(dR)

(ℓB)

(dR)

A

(O)

(dB)

caecal
diverticulum

stomach
(dR)

(dB)

(dR)

A

(ℓB)

(O)

(ℓB)

stomach
(dR)

(dR)

(O)

(ℓB)

direction of
descent (dB)

STAGE 16 STAGE 17 WEEK 12

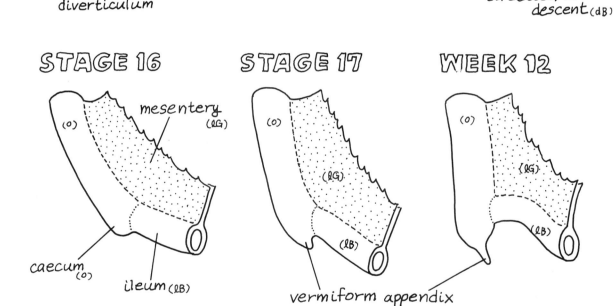

mesentery
(ℓG)

(O)

caecum
(O)

ileum (ℓB)

(O)

(ℓG)

(ℓB)

vermiform appendix

(O)

(ℓG)

(ℓB)

NEONATE ADULT

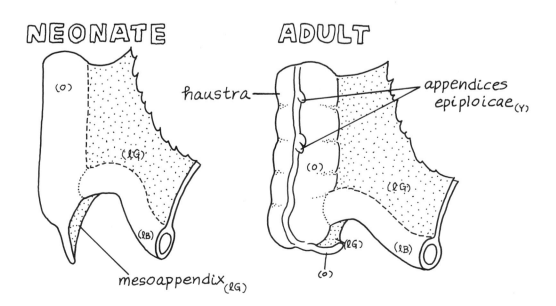

(O)

(ℓG)

mesoappendix (ℓG)

haustra

(O)

(ℓG)

(O)

appendices
epiploicae (Y)

(ℓG)

(ℓB)

81. Hindgut: Partition of Cloaca

The early hindgut ends as an expanded chamber called the cloaca ('sewer'). The cloacal membrane forms when the endoderm lining the cloaca contacts the ectoderm of the proctodeum or anal pit. This membrane is surrounded by a circular cloacal sphincter.

In Week 7, a wedge of tissue called the urorectal septum grows into and divides the cloaca, the cloacal membrane and the cloacal sphincter into two main regions. The urogenital sinus is situated ventrally, and the rectum and anal canal dorsally.

81. HINDGUT : PARTITION OF CLOACA

STAGE 13

✛(R) : URORECTAL SEPTUM(dR)
▷(dB) : CLOACAL MEMBRANE(dG)

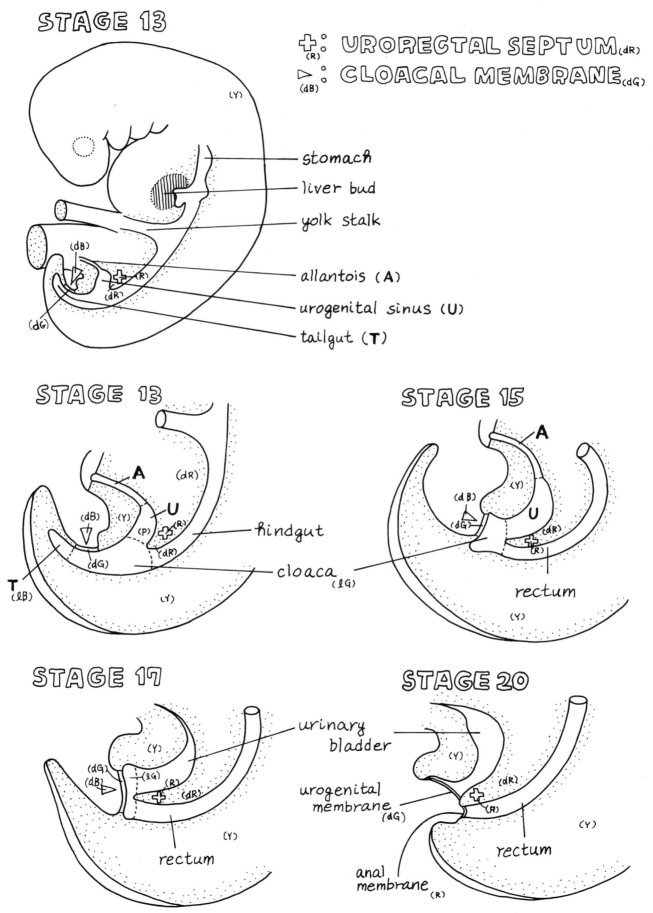

(Y)

stomach
liver bud
yolk stalk

(dB)
✛(R)
(dR)
(dG)

allantois (A)
urogenital sinus (U)
tailgut (T)

STAGE 13

A
(dR)
(dB)
(Y)
U
(P)
✛(R)
(dR)
(dG)
T
(ℓB)
(Y)

hindgut

cloaca
(ℓG)

STAGE 15

A
(dB)
(Y)
U
(dG)
(dR)
✛(R)

rectum
(Y)

STAGE 17

(Y)
(dG)
(dB)
(ℓG)
(R)
✛
(dR)

rectum
(Y)

urinary
bladder

STAGE 20

(Y)
(dR)
✛
(R)

urogenital
membrane
(dG)

rectum
(Y)

anal
membrane (R)

213

82. Hindgut: Anal Canal

As the urorectal septum grows into the cloaca, it divides it into the urogenital sinus ventrally, and the rectum and anal canal dorsally. The urorectal septum then fuses with the cloacal membrane dividing it into an urogenital membrane and an anal membrane. The surrounding sphincter is divided into the sphincter of the urogenital sinus and an external anal sphincter.

In the adult, the site of the urorectal septum fusing with the cloacal membrane is marked by a fibromuscular node called the central perineal tendon (or perineal body). In the mother, this site is vulnerable during childbirth, as the great pressure exerted can tear the muscles which converge and insert here.

The anal membrane ruptures during Week 8, which allows continuity between the amniotic cavity and the anal canal. The approximate site of this membrane can be located in the adult as the pectinate line. The superior two-thirds of the anal canal above the pectinate line is derived from hindgut and the inferior one-third below it from the proctodeum. The blood supply, lymphatic drainage and nerve supply of the anal canal reflect these two origins.

Anomalies of the Anal Canal

Most anorectal malformations are due to the anomalous development of the urorectal septum. Anal agenesis with or without a fistula may occur either as a high or low anorectal anomaly.

82. HINDGUT : ANAL CANAL

STAGE 16

WEEK 8

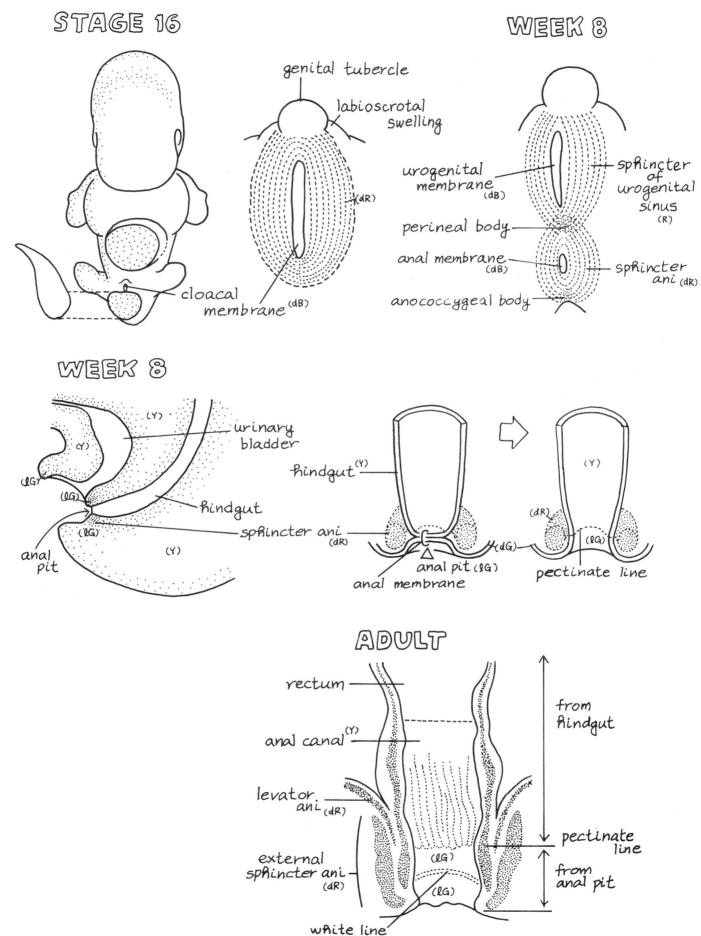

genital tubercle

labioscrotal swelling

(dR)

cloacal membrane (dB)

urogenital membrane (dB)

sphincter of urogenital sinus (R)

perineal body

anal membrane (dB)

sphincter ani (dR)

anococcygeal body

WEEK 8

(Y)

(Y)

urinary bladder

(lG)

(lG)

hindgut

(lG)

sphincter ani (dR)

anal pit

(Y)

hindgut (Y)

sphincter ani (dR)

anal pit (lG)

anal membrane

(dG)

(dR)

(Y)

(lG)

pectinate line

ADULT

rectum

anal canal (Y)

levator ani (dR)

external sphincter ani (dR)

white line

(lG)

(lG)

from hindgut

pectinate line

from anal pit

UROGENITAL SYSTEM

83. Kidneys: Pronephros

Urogenital System

The urinary system and reproductive system are closely related developmentally and anatomically and are referred to as the urogenital (urinary and reproductive) system. Both systems are derivatives of a longitudinal ridge of intermediate mesoderm called the urogenital ridge. This ridge has two main regions: a nephrogenic cord which gives rise to the urinary system and the gonadal ridge which gives rise to the genital system.

Three successive sets of kidneys and their associated ducts develop in the human: the pronephros, mesonephros and metanephros. The first and second sets largely disappear while the metanephros will form the adult kidney.

Pronephros

The pronephros (pleural: pronephroi) appears in Week 4 as rudimentary groups of cells in the cervical region. While the pronephroi are transitory and degenerate, their two ducts, which open into the cloaca, will become the ducts of the mesonephros.

UROGENITAL SYSTEM
83. KIDNEYS: PRONEPHROS

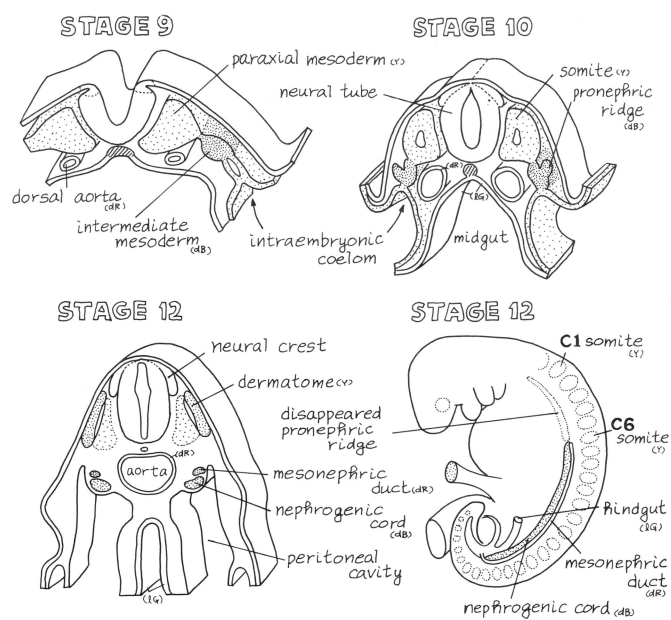

STAGE 9

paraxial mesoderm (Y)

dorsal aorta (dR)

intermediate mesoderm (dB)

STAGE 10

neural tube

somite (Y)
pronephric ridge (dB)

intraembryonic coelom

midgut

STAGE 12

neural crest

dermatome (Y)

disappeared pronephric ridge

mesonephric duct (dR)

nephrogenic cord (dB)

peritoneal cavity

aorta (dR)

(lG)

STAGE 12

C1 somite (Y)

C6 somite (Y)

hindgut (lG)

mesonephric duct (dR)

nephrogenic cord (dB)

84. Kidneys: Mesonephros

The mesonephros (pleural: mesonephroi) is the second stage of kidney development and contains functional renal tissue.

In Week 4, the mesonephros appears caudal to the pronephros. This new kidney utilises the adjacent pronephric duct, which is now renamed the mesonephric duct. The mesonephroi are large organs which function until their activity is replaced by that of the third set of kidneys the metanephros.

The mesonephroi are simple organs composed of glomeruli and tubules. Between Weeks 5–11, the nephrogenic cords become canalised and form mesonephric vesicles. Each vesicle forms an 'S' shaped mesonephric tubule which joins to the mesonephric duct. The medial end of the tubule then becomes invaginated by a cluster of capillaries from the aorta. Each capillary is a simple glomerulus and the medial end of the tubule forms Bowman's capsule (or glomerular capsule). Blood from the glomerulus passes into a capillary plexus and thence to the posterior cardinal vein and sub-cardinal vein system. The most cephalic tubules progressively degenerate while more new tubules form at caudal levels. A fairly constant number of tubules is present between Weeks 4–9. When the third set of kidneys are established, the mesonephroi and their blood supply rapidly involute. Some of the tubules and ducts persist as the paradidymis in the male and as the paroophoron and epoophoron in the female (see **98**. Early Female and Male Duct Systems).

84. KIDNEYS : MESONEPHROS

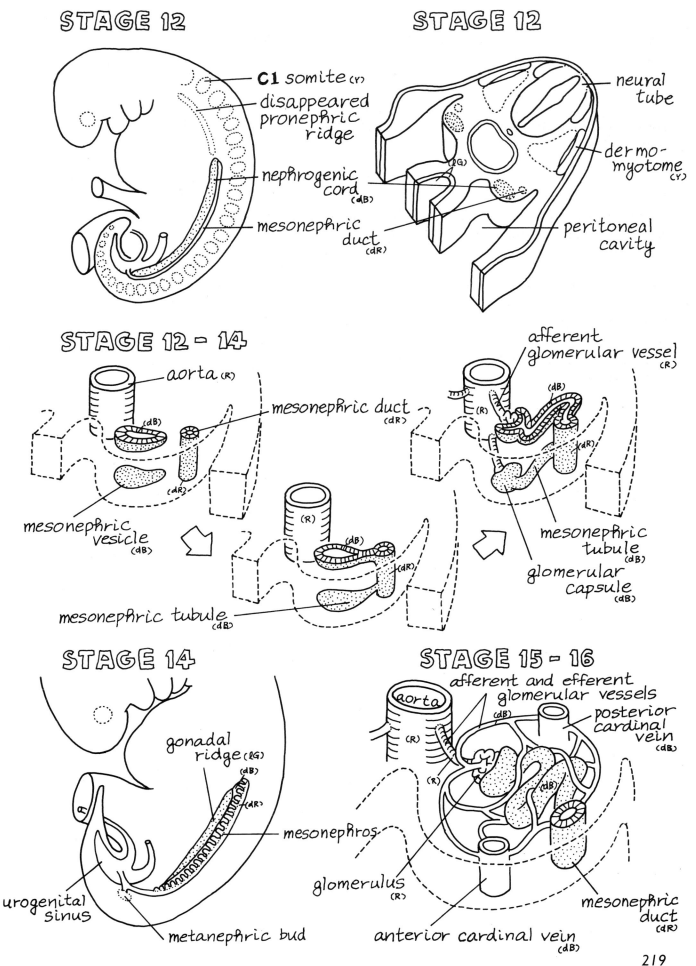

STAGE 12

C1 somite (r)

disappeared pronephric ridge

nephrogenic cord (dB)

mesonephric duct (dR)

STAGE 12

neural tube

dermo-myotome (Y)

(G)

peritoneal cavity

STAGE 12 - 14

aorta (R)

(dB)

mesonephric duct (dR)

(dR)

mesonephric vesicle (dB)

(R)

(dB)

(dR)

mesonephric tubule (dB)

afferent glomerular vessel (R)

(dB)

(R)

(dR)

mesonephric tubule (dB)

glomerular capsule (dB)

STAGE 14

gonadal ridge (lG)

(dB)

(dR)

mesonephros

urogenital sinus

metanephric bud

STAGE 15 - 16

afferent and efferent glomerular vessels (dB)

posterior cardinal vein (dB)

aorta

(R)

(R)

(dB)

glomerulus (R)

mesonephric duct (dR)

anterior cardinal vein (dB)

85. Kidneys: Metanephros

The third set of kidneys, the metanephroi, appears in Week 5 (Stages 13–14), and will give rise to the adult kidneys. Each of these permanent kidneys arises from two primordia: the metanephric diverticulum (or ureteric bud) and the metanephric mesoderm.

The metanephric diverticulum first appears as a dorsal bud from the mesonephric duct near its entrance into the cloaca. This bud grows into the adjacent metanephric mesoderm inducing it to form the metanephric mass or cap over the bud. The bud will give rise to the collecting system: ureter, renal pelvis, calyces and collecting tubules. The collecting tubules divide repeatedly. They successively form the major calyces, minor calyces, and finally the permanent collecting tubules. The metanephric mesenchyme adjacent to the collecting tubules is induced to form metanephric vesicles and tubules. Each metanephric tubule then connects to the adjacent collecting tubule. Bowman's capsules are formed as glomeruli invaginate the ends of the metanephric or renal tubules.

In summary, this means that the distal convoluted tubule, loop of Henle, proximal convoluted tubule and renal corpuscle (Bowman's capsule and glomerulus) arise from the metanephric mesoderm, whilst the collecting system arises from the metanephric diverticulum.

Urine formation begins around Weeks 11–13.

85. KIDNEYS: METANEPHROS
STAGE 13 - 14

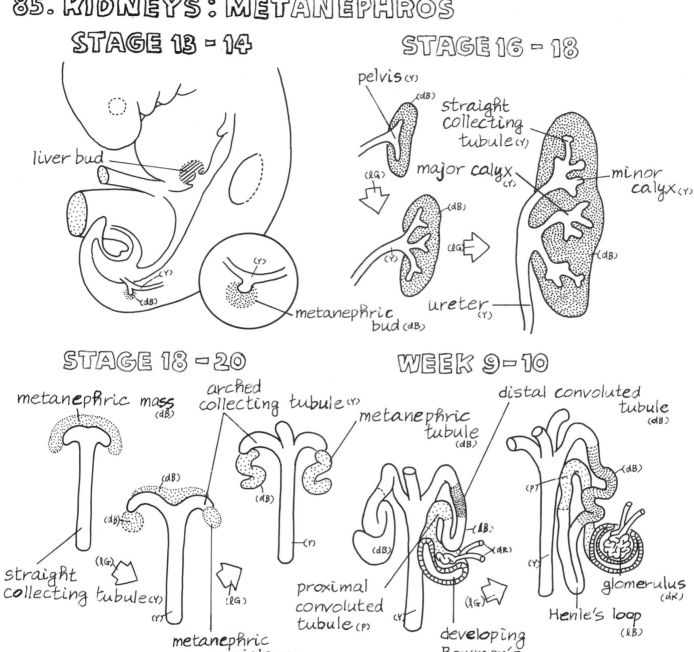

STAGE 16 - 18

liver bud

metanephric bud (dB)

pelvis (Y)
(dB)
straight collecting tubule (Y)
(lG)
major calyx (Y)
minor calyx (Y)
(dB)
(lG)
(Y)
ureter (Y)
(dB)

STAGE 18 - 20

metanephric mass (dB)

arched collecting tubule (Y)

metanephric tubule (dB)

straight collecting tubule (Y)

(dB)
(lG)
(Y)

metanephric vesicle (dB)

(dB)
(Y)

WEEK 9 - 10

distal convoluted tubule (dB)

proximal convoluted tubule (P)

developing Bowman's capsule

(dB)
(P)
(lG)
(Y)
(lB)
(dR)

metanephric tubule (dB)

distal convoluted tubule (dB)
(dB)
(P)
(Y)

glomerulus (dR)

Henle's loop (lB)

86. Fetal Kidneys

By Week 10, the fetal metanephric kidneys have migrated into the abdominal cavity. The kidneys have a slightly lobulated surface. At this stage glomeruli form and a small number of early nephrons are found.

By Week 23, the subdivision of the renal pelvis is complete. The medulla and cortex are almost fully developed by the eighth month.

The fetal and newborn kidneys are lobulated reflecting the 5–25 renal lobes seen during development. The kidney normally does not have a smooth surface until 4–5 years after birth.

The fetal kidneys begin to function at 3 months and contribute urine to the amniotic fluid (Week 12). Their functioning is assessed by bladder function on ultrasound scans. *In utero* the placenta is responsible for eliminating fetal waste products.

Most of the glomeruli and convoluted tubules appear by the time of birth. Some additional ones differentiate from mesenchyme in the months after birth. Future renal growth is by enlargement of existing renal tissue.

Although glomeruli in the neonate appear similar in structure to those of the adult, their filtration rates are reduced until 6 weeks of age.

86. FETAL KIDNEYS

WEEK 10

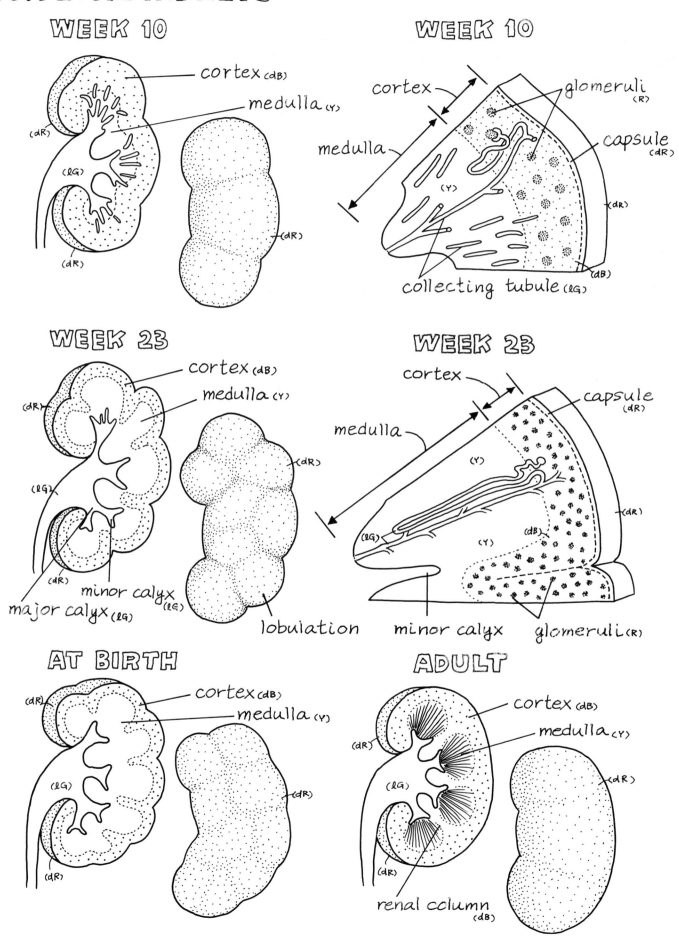

cortex (dB)

medulla (Y)

(dR)

(lG)

(dR)

WEEK 10

cortex

medulla

(Y)

glomeruli (R)

capsule (dR)

(dR)

(dB)

collecting tubule (lG)

WEEK 23

cortex (dB)

medulla (Y)

(dR)

(lG)

(dR)

major calyx (lG)

minor calyx (lG)

lobulation

WEEK 23

cortex

medulla

capsule (dR)

(Y)

(lG)

(dB)

(dR)

(Y)

minor calyx

glomeruli (R)

AT BIRTH

cortex (dB)

medulla (Y)

(dR)

(lG)

(dR)

(dR)

ADULT

cortex (dB)

medulla (Y)

(dR)

(lG)

(dR)

(dR)

renal column (dB)

87. Kidneys: Positional Changes

The metanephric kidneys initially develop close together in the pelvic region and come to assume a more cephalic position next to the suprarenal glands in Week 9. Their migration is actually a 'relative' movement caused by the rapid growth of the embryo's body caudal to the kidneys. At this time three other processes occur: the hilum of the kidney which originally faces ventrally, rotates through 90° to face the midline, the blood supply changes (see below), and the ureters increase in length.

87. KIDNEYS: POSITIONAL CHANGES

STAGE 14

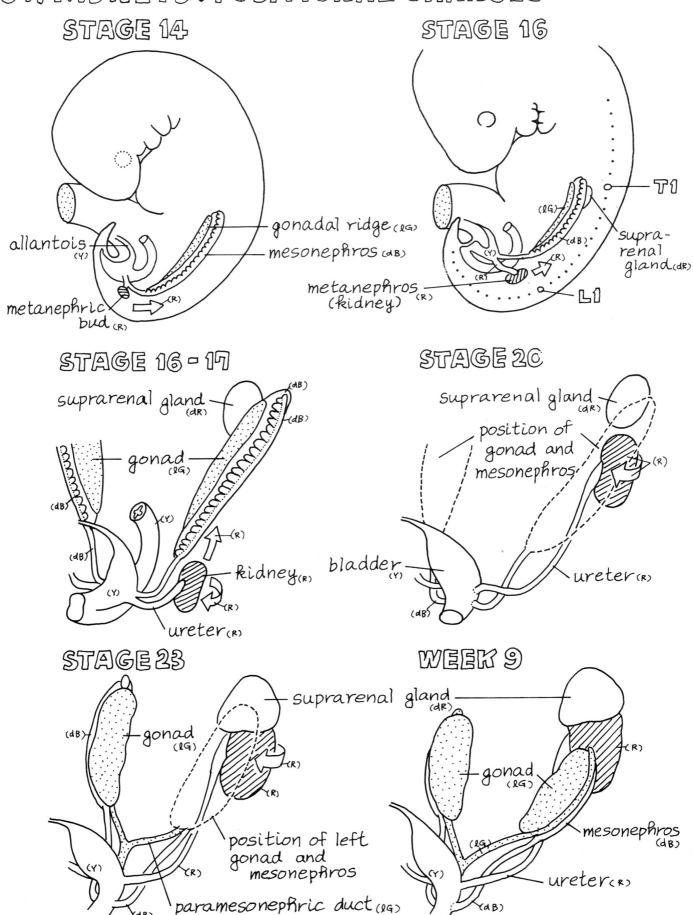

allantois (Y)

gonadal ridge (lG)

mesonephros (dB)

metanephric bud (R)

STAGE 16

(lG)

(dB)

(Y)

(R)

(R)

T1

supra-renal gland (dR)

metanephros (kidney) (R)

L1

STAGE 16-17

suprarenal gland (dR)

(dB)

(dB)

gonad (lG)

(dB)

(Y)

(dB)

(R)

kidney (R)

(Y)

(R)

ureter (R)

STAGE 20

suprarenal gland (dR)

position of gonad and mesonephros

(R)

bladder (Y)

(dB)

ureter (R)

STAGE 23

(dB)

gonad (lG)

suprarenal gland (dR)

(R)

(R)

(Y)

(R)

position of left gonad and mesonephros

paramesonephric duct (lG)

(dB)

WEEK 9

suprarenal gland (dR)

(R)

gonad (lG)

mesonephros (dB)

(lG)

(Y)

ureter (R)

(dB)

225

Blood Supply

Initially each kidney is supplied by a branch from the common iliac artery. Then as the kidney ascends, a new artery (renal artery) forms from the aorta to supply the kidney in its new position and the inferior branches degenerate and disappear.

Anomalies of Migration

The kidneys may be left in an ectopic position because of partial migration and the hilum may not have rotated medially. These kidneys are supplied by nearby blood vessels rather than the definitive renal artery.

Supernumerary blood vessels are common, more often arteries than veins. 'Horseshoe' kidneys arise if migration is prevented by the root of the inferior mesenteric artery. Such kidneys usually lie in the hypogastrium near the lumbar vertebrae and are fused.

WEEK 12 - 13 (MALE)

DEVELOPING BLOOD SUPPLY

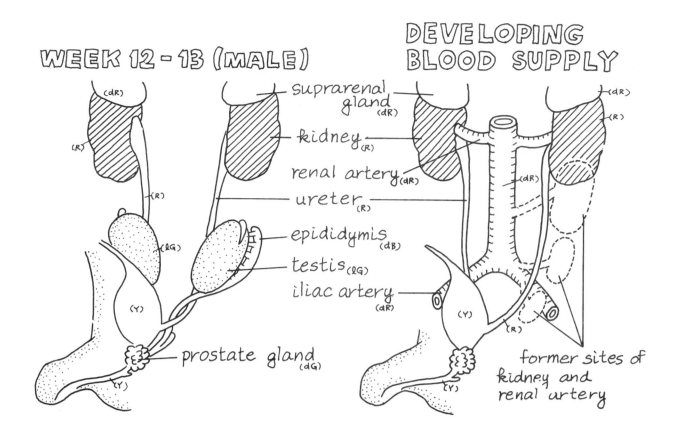

suprarenal gland (dR)

kidney (R)

renal artery (dR)

ureter (R)

epididymis (dB)

testis (lG)

iliac artery (dR)

prostate gland (dG)

former sites of kidney and renal artery

88. Suprarenal Glands (Adrenals)

The primordia of the suprarenal glands first appear in Week 6 near the cephalic end of the mesonephros. Mesenchyme from the posterior abdominal wall forms the fetal cortex, while nearby neural crest cells migrate from a sympathetic ganglion to form the medulla.

Initially the medulla is a mass of cells on the medial aspect of the fetal cortex (Weeks 7–8). Gradually as the cortex grows and enlarges, it surrounds and envelopes the medulla (Weeks 8–10). More mesenchyme cells from the posterior abdominal wall enclose the fetal cortex. Eventually this new mesenchyme layer will form the permanent cortex (Weeks 10–14), and the medulla will form the secretory cells of the medulla.

By Week 30, two more layers of the fetal cortex differentiate to form the zona glomerulosa and the zona fasciculata. By birth the fetal cortex is beginning to regress and ultimately disappears by one postnatal year. The zona reticularis of the cortex normally appears by the end of year three postnatally.

The adrenal gland is relatively large in the fetus due to the large fetal cortex which regresses after birth.

Anomalies of the Suprarenals

Anencephalic infants lacking a pituitary are deficient in adrenocorticotrophic hormone (ACTH) and develop hypoplastic suprarenal glands.

88. SUPRARENAL GLANDS (ADRENALS)

STAGE 16

STAGE 16

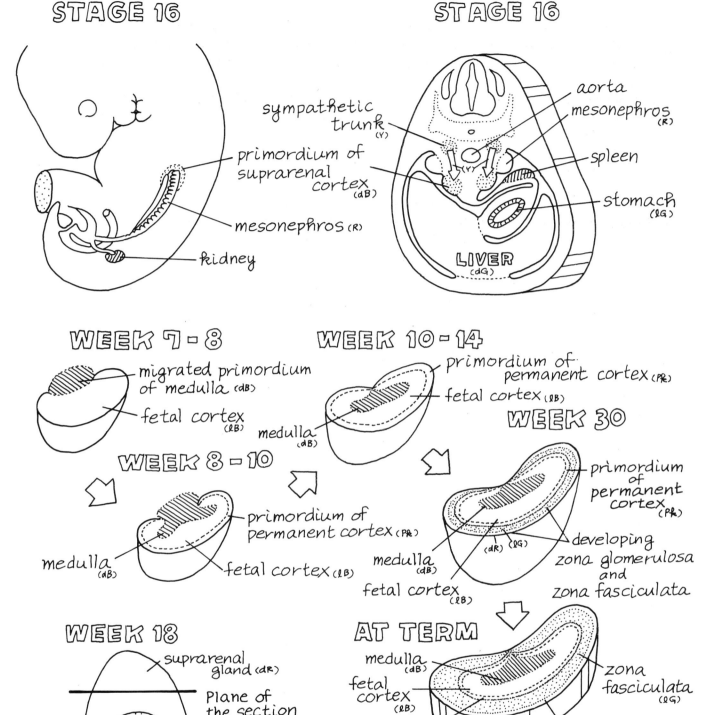

sympathetic trunk (Y)

primordium of suprarenal cortex (dB)

mesonephros (R)

kidney

aorta

mesonephros (R)

spleen

stomach (lG)

LIVER (dG)

WEEK 7 - 8

migrated primordium of medulla (dB)

fetal cortex (lB)

WEEK 10 - 14

primordium of permanent cortex (PR)

fetal cortex (lB)

medulla (dB)

WEEK 8 - 10

medulla (dB)

primordium of permanent cortex (PR)

fetal cortex (lB)

WEEK 30

primordium of permanent cortex (PR)

developing zona glomerulosa and zona fasciculata

medulla (dB)

fetal cortex (lB)

(dR) (lG)

WEEK 18

suprarenal gland (dR)

Plane of the section

kidney (B)

AT TERM

medulla (dB)

fetal cortex (lB)

primordium of permanent cortex (PR)

zona fasciculata (lG)

zona glomerulosa (dR)

after 1 YEAR

medulla (dB)

developing zona reticularis (R)

(dR) (lG)

medulla (dB)

disappearing fetal cortex (lB)

zona fasciculata (lG)

primordium of permanent cortex (PR)

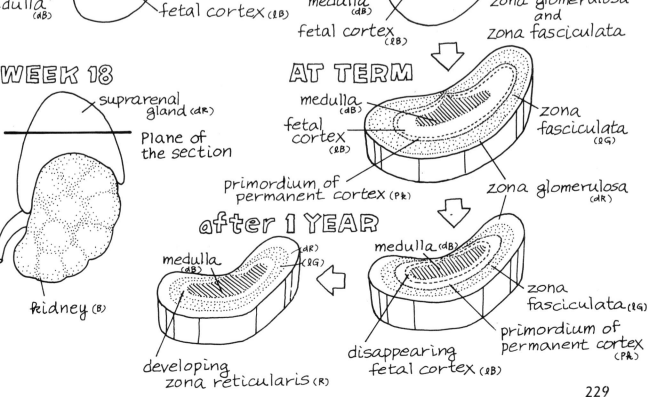

89. Ureters

The ureters are derivatives of the mesenchymal metanephric diverticula (or ureteric buds). As each metanephric diverticulum grows into the adjacent metanephric mesoderm, it induces the mesoderm to form the metanephric mass or cap over the end of the diverticulum.

The stalk of the metanephric diverticulum will form the ureter, and where the metanephric mass surrounds it, the future ureter is expanded to form the renal pelvis.

The ureters initially are diverticula of the mesonephric ducts, but as each duct is gradually incorporated into the bladder in the region of the trigone, so are the ureters. They ultimately enter the wall of the bladder at an angle which helps prevent the reflux of urine. Their cephalic ends assume their adult position as the developing kidneys undergo their relative ascent from the pelvic region to their final position on the posterior abdominal wall.

Anomalies of the Ureter

The metanephric diverticulum may divide partially to form a bifid ureter or completely to form two separate ureters.

89. URETERS

STAGE 14

gonad

mesonephros

metanephros (kidney) (dR)

(dB)

(Y)

STAGE 14 - 16

allantois (Y)

cloacal membrane (B)

mesonephric duct (lG)

urogenital sinus (Y)

ureter (dR)

(dB)

hindgut (rectum)

(Y)

(lG)

(dB)

(lG)

ureter (dR)

(dR)

STAGE 18 - 19

allantois (dG)

mesonephric duct (lG)

urinary bladder (Y)

ureter (dR)

developing urethra (R)

rectum (dB)

(Y)

(lG)

STAGE 22

(dG)

(Y)

ureter (dR)

(lG)

STAGE 23

(dG)

ureter (dR)

(lG)

(Y)

(R)

WEEK 11 - 12 (♂)

urachus (dG) (allantois)

ureter (dR)

ductus deferens (mesonephric duct) (lG)

prostate gland (o)

rectum

urethra (R)

(Y)

(o)

(o)

WEEK 11 - 12 (♂)

BLADDER (Y)

ureter (dR)

prostate gland (o)

(Pk)

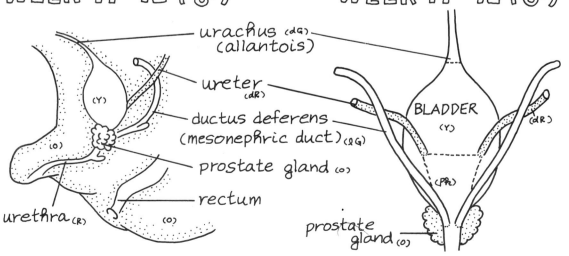

90. Urinary Bladder

The bladder forms from the urogenital sinus. It is continuous with the allantois above and with the phallus below. The transitional epithelium lining the entire bladder (including the trigone region) is derived from the endoderm of the urogenital sinus. The muscular layers are derivatives of the surrounding splanchnic mesenchyme.

Two pairs of vessels enter the dorsal bladder wall on each side: the metanephric duct (future ureter) and the mesonephric duct. As the bladder enlarges the caudal ends of the ducts are incorporated into the bladder wall. This region of incorporation is known as the trigone and is identifiable in the adult as a smooth, triangular area on the dorsal wall. Cells from the ducts also contribute to the connective tissue of the mucosa.

Initially the two vessels on each side enter the bladder in close proximity. However, they soon become separated as the ureters move superolaterally and pass through the bladder wall more obliquely. This movement superolaterally is linked with the 'relative ascent' of the kidneys.

The two mesonephric ducts come to lie close together. In the female their caudal ends degenerate, while in the male they form the ejaculatory ducts which enter the prostatic urethra.

At the apex of the bladder, the allantois involutes and thickens to form a tube, the urachus. The urachus remains attached distally to the umbilicus and the two umbilical arteries pass to the umbilical cord in its margins. After birth, the urachus forms the fibrous median umbilical ligament. The proximal parts of the umbilical arteries form the superior vesical arteries supplying the bladder and the distal parts form the medial umbilical ligaments.

The fetal bladder normally fills and empties every 40–60 minutes and this can be visualised by ultrasound scanning. An abnormal emptying pattern is often associated with anomalies of the urinary system. The fetal and neonatal bladder is normally an abdominal organ which gradually becomes a pelvic organ during and after puberty.

Anomalies of the Bladder

In exstrophy of the bladder, both the anterior bladder wall and part of the abdominal wall have ruptured because of failure of the formation of the abdominal musculature.

90. URINARY BLADDER

STAGE 13

metanephric bud (dR)

STAGE 14 - 16

mesonephric duct (lG)

allantois (Y)

cloacal membrane (dB)

(Y)

(R)

(dB)

ureter (dR)

metanephros (kidney) (dR)

STAGE 18

mesonephric duct (lG)

urinary bladder (Y)

ureter (dR)

rectum (dB)

STAGE 19 - 21

allantois (Y)

urinary bladder (Y)

(R)

(lG)

(dR)

future trigone

(Y)

STAGE 23

allantois (Y)

(Y)

(lG)

ureter (dR)

trigone

orifice of fused paramesonephric duct

ADULT

♀ ♂

urachus (Y)

(Y)

(lG)

trigone

seminal vesicle (dB)

(Y)

(lG)

prostate gland (dR)

233

91. Urethra

In Weeks 4–7, the urorectal septum divides the cloaca into the urogenital sinus and the rectum. The endodermal urogenital sinus extends to the base of the phallus as the urethral groove. The epithelium of the female urethra is completely derived from the endodermal urogenital sinus. Most of the epithelium of the male urethra arises from the endoderm from the urogenital sinus with a contribution from the surface ectoderm. The smooth muscle and connective tissue in both male and female forms from adjacent splanchnic mesenchyme. As the urogenital folds fuse in Weeks 9–12, the urethral groove forms a tube which becomes the whole urethra in the female and forms part of the urethra in the male.

The urethra in the male also has an ectodermal contribution, as well as the endodermal contribution from the urethral groove. A cellular cord of ectoderm called the glandular plate grows into the developing glans penis. The cellular cord then connects to the developing spongy urethra and becomes canalised, so allowing the urethra to open onto the tip of the glans.

91. URETHRA

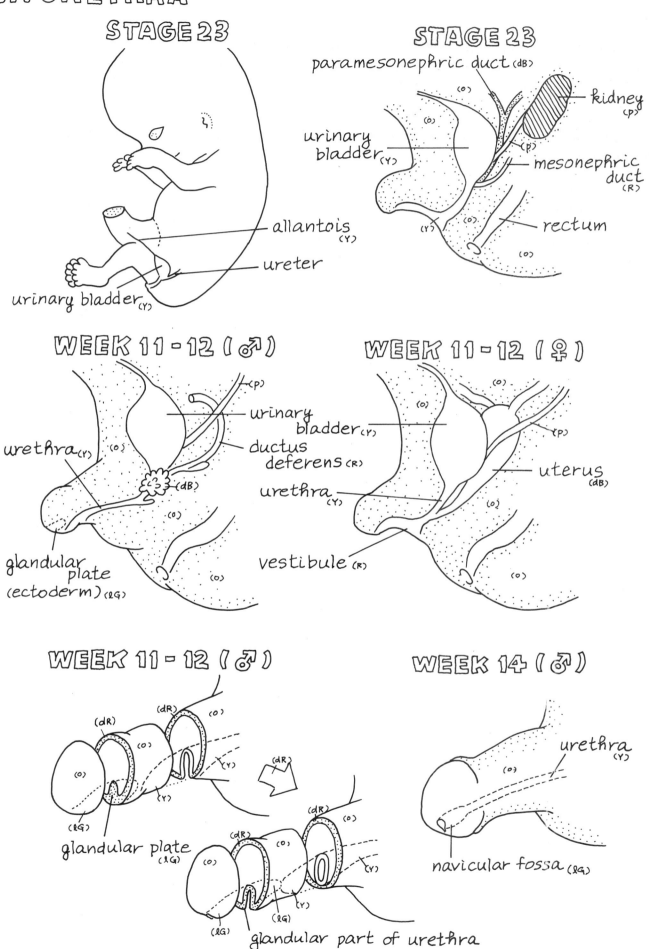

STAGE 23

allantois (Y)

ureter

urinary bladder (Y)

STAGE 23

paramesonephric duct (dB)

kidney (P)

urinary bladder (Y)

mesonephric duct (R)

rectum

WEEK 11-12 (♂)

urinary bladder (Y)

ductus deferens (R)

urethra (Y)

glandular plate (ectoderm) (lG)

WEEK 11-12 (♀)

urinary bladder (Y)

uterus (dB)

urethra (Y)

vestibule (R)

WEEK 11-12 (♂)

glandular plate (lG)

glandular part of urethra

WEEK 14 (♂)

urethra (Y)

navicular fossa (lG)

92. Prostate Gland

The prostate gland arises toward the end of the third month as solid buds grow out from the prostatic urethral epithelium into adjacent mesenchyme. The endoderm gives rise to the glandular epithelium and the mesenchyme gives rise to smooth muscle fibres and connective tissue.

A diverticulum that opens into the prostatic urethra is called the prostatic utricle and is homologous to the vagina.

By the fourth month, as many as 50 prostatic outgrowths may be present and the buds begin to canalise to form lumina.

By the fifth month, the tissue surrounding the prostatic utricle forms cysts and the capsule differentiates. A glycogen-rich secretion appears in the ducts of the gland during the ninth month.

92. PROSTATE GLAND

WEEK 11-12

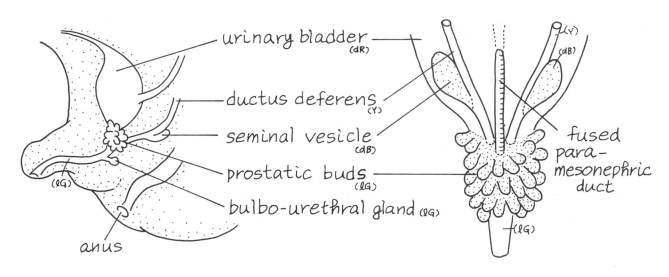

WEEK 11-12

urinary bladder — (dR)

ductus deferens (Y)

seminal vesicle (dB)

prostatic buds (lG)

bulbo-urethral gland (lG)

anus

(lG)

fused para-mesonephric duct

(Y) (dB)

(lG)

WEEK 16

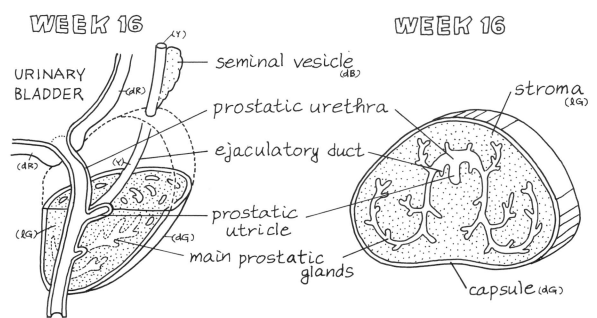

WEEK 16

(Y)

URINARY BLADDER

(dR)

(dR)

(lG)

(Y)

(dG)

seminal vesicle (dB)

prostatic urethra

ejaculatory duct

prostatic utricle

main prostatic glands

stroma (lG)

capsule (dG)

93. Urachus

The bladder is initially continuous with the allantois which extends into the umbilical cord. Though the extraembryonic portion of the allantois degenerates during the second month, the intra-abdominal portion involutes to form a tube called the urachus. The urachus is attached to the umbilicus and to the apex of the bladder. On either side of the urachus lies an umbilical artery.

In the adult, the fibrous urachus forms the median umbilical ligament and the two fibrosed umbilical arteries form the two medial umbilical ligaments.

Anomalies of the Urachus

An urachal fistula forms if the entire urachus remains patent and urine escapes from its orifice in the umbilicus. If the urachus remains patent inferiorly, it may dilate and form an urachal sinus opening into the bladder. If the urachus remains patent superiorly, it may dilate and form an urachal sinus opening at the umbilicus. Urachal cysts may form if remnants of the lumen persist in the urachus.

93. URACHUS

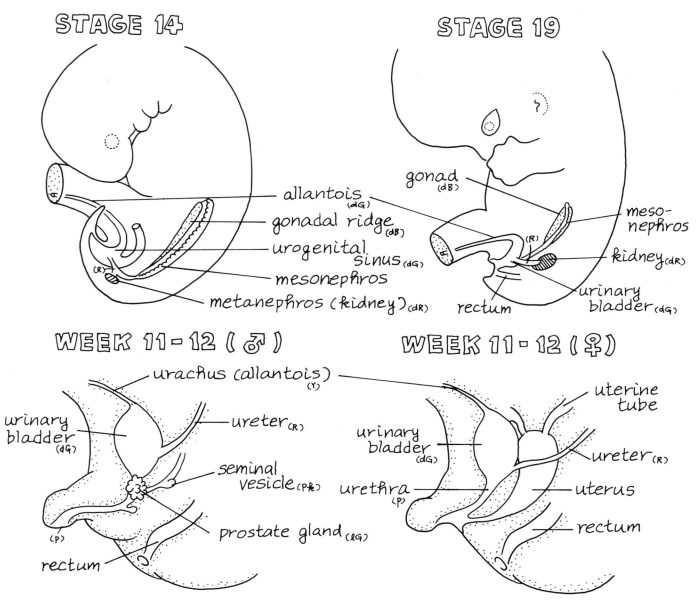

STAGE 14

STAGE 19

allantois (dG)
gonadal ridge (dB)
urogenital sinus (dG)
mesonephros
metanephros (kidney) (dR)

gonad (dB)
meso-nephros
kidney (dR)
rectum
urinary bladder (dG)

WEEK 11-12 (♂)

urachus (allantois) (Y)
urinary bladder (dG)
ureter (R)
seminal vesicle (P*)
prostate gland (lG)
rectum
(P)

WEEK 11-12 (♀)

uterine tube
urinary bladder (dG)
ureter (R)
urethra (P)
uterus
rectum

MALFORMATIONS OF THE URACHUS

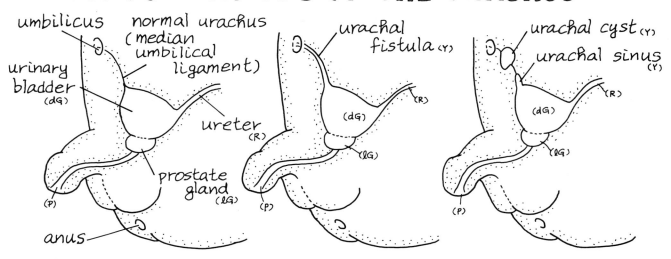

umbilicus
normal urachus (median umbilical ligament)
urinary bladder (dG)
ureter (R)
prostate gland (lG)
anus
(P)

urachal fistula (Y)
(dG)
(R)
(lG)
(P)

urachal cyst (Y)
urachal sinus (Y)
(dG)
(R)
(lG)
(P)

94. Early Gonads

The primordial germ cells are first identifiable in the endoderm of the yolk sac near the allantois.

As the yolk sac is incorporated into the embryo during the formation of the body folds, the primordial germ cells enter the abdomen and migrate on the dorsal gut mesentery to the gonadal ridges. Upon reaching the ridges, they migrate into the mesenchyme and form part of the primary sex cords. Although the genetic sex of the embryo is determined at fertilisation, the gonads in both sexes appear to be identical until Week 7 ('indifferent' gonads). The normal female sex chromosome complement is XX and the normal male is XY. There are several abnormalities of the female including XO and XXX and of the male XXY and XYY. Trisomy, tetrasomy and pentasomy of the sex chromosomes may occur in both sexes.

The presence or absence of a Y chromosome will determine whether the indifferent gonads differentiate into male or female gonads

94. EARLY GONADS
STAGE 11

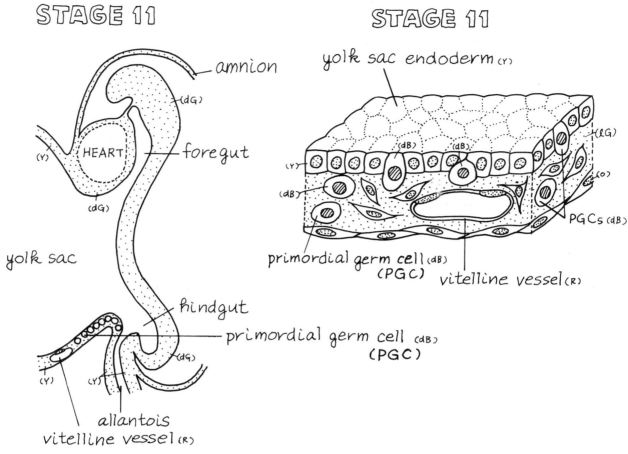

amnion

(dG)

HEART

(Y)

foregut

(dG)

yolk sac

hindgut

primordial germ cell (dB)
(PGC)

(dG)

(Y)

(Y)

allantois

vitelline vessel (R)

STAGE 11

yolk sac endoderm (Y)

(dB)   (dB)

(Y)

(dB)

(ℓG)

(O)

PGCs (dB)

primordial germ cell (dB)
(PGC)

vitelline vessel (R)

STAGE 14

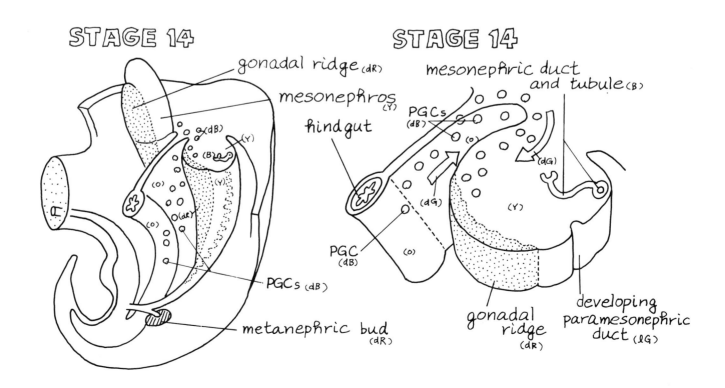

gonadal ridge (dR)

mesonephros (Y)

(dB)

(Y)

(B)

(O)

(Y)

O (dR)

(O)

PGCs (dB)

metanephric bud (dR)

STAGE 14

mesonephric duct
and tubule (B)

PGCs (dB)

hindgut

(O)

(dG)

(dG)

(Y)

PGC (dB)

(O)

gonadal ridge (dR)

developing paramesonephric duct (ℓG)

95. Development of the Ovaries

The primordial germ cells of female embryos migrate to the gonadal ridge from the yolk sac. Primary sex cords grow into the medulla of the developing ovary. The cords are never prominent and although they form a rete ovarii, this structure and the cords normally degenerate.

Later the secondary sex cords (called cortical cords) grow from the surface epithelium into the medulla where they incorporate the primordial germ cells. Each germ cell is surrounded by a layer of flattened cells from its cortical cord. As the cortical cords disperse, the germ cells which by now have formed oogonia, are surrounded by flattened cells and form primordial follicles. These primordial follicles repeatedly divide and no further oogonia are formed postnatally. The flattened cells around the oogonia become cuboidal and the follicles are now known as primary follicles. These will develop further at puberty.

As the mesonephroi regress, each ovary is suspended by its own mesentery, the mesovarium. The surface epithelium is separated from the cortex and the primary follicles, as a fibrous layer (the tunica albuginea) forms between the two layers.

95. DEVELOPMENT OF THE OVARIES

STAGE 14

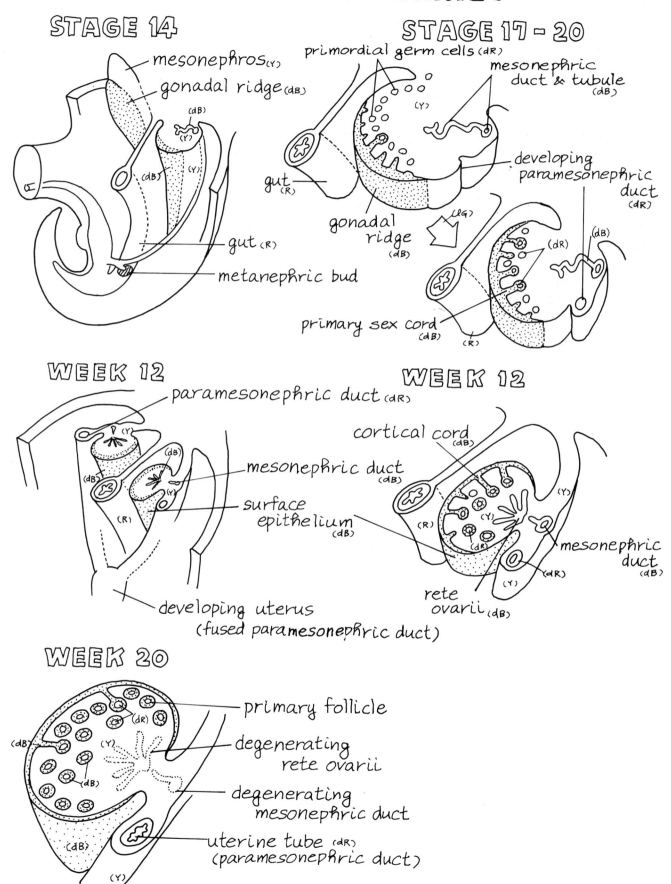

mesonephros (Y)

gonadal ridge (dB)

(dB)
(Y)

(dB) (Y)

gut (R)

metanephric bud

STAGE 17 - 20

primordial germ cells (dR)

mesonephric duct & tubule (dB)

(Y)

gut (R)

developing paramesonephric duct (dR)

gonadal ridge (dB)

(dR)

(dB)

primary sex cord (dB)

(R)

WEEK 12

paramesonephric duct (dR)

(Y)

(dB)

(dB)

(Y)

(R)

mesonephric duct (dB)

surface epithelium (dB)

developing uterus
(fused paramesonephric duct)

WEEK 12

cortical cord (dB)

(Y)

(R)

(Y)

(dR)

mesonephric duct (dB)

(dR)

(Y)

rete ovarii (dB)

WEEK 20

(dB)

(dR)

(Y)

(dB)

(dB)

(Y)

primary follicle

degenerating rete ovarii

degenerating mesonephric duct

uterine tube (dR)
(paramesonephric duct)

243

96. Uterine Tubes, Uterus and Vagina

The uterine tubes, uterus and superior part of the vagina develop from the paramesonephric (Mullerian) ducts.

The paramesonephric ducts arise on the lateral aspects of the mesonephroi. As the mesodermal epithelium invaginates, a tube is formed where the edges of the invagination fuse. The open cranial ends of the tube are funnel-shaped and continuous with the peritoneal cavity. This region will form the uterine tubes. The caudal ends fuse in the median plane and form the uterovaginal primordium. This primordium projects into the urogenital sinus. Its position is marked on the internal aspect of the urogenital sinus as the sinus tubercle. When the uterovaginal primordium contacts the urogenital sinus, it induces two endodermal outgrowths called the sinovaginal bulbs. These soon fuse and extend from the urogenital sinus up to the uterovaginal primordium. This solid vaginal plate obliterates the lumen. Later, the centre will break down to re-establish the lumen. The peripheral cells become the vaginal epithelium.

The myometrium (muscle layer) of the uterovaginal primordium and its endometrial stroma are derivatives of adjacent mesenchyme.

The superior part of the vagina is derived from the uterovaginal primordium, while the inferior part forms from the urogenital sinus. The hymen separates the superior from the inferior part of the vagina until late fetal life. It usually ruptures in the perinatal period leaving a thin layer of mucous membrane around the perimeter of the vaginal lumen.

The urethral and paraurethral glands develop when buds from the urethra grow into the adjacent mesenchyme. The greater vestibular glands (of Bartholin) develop from outgrowths of the urogenital sinus.

Studies in experimental animals show that removal of the ovaries has no effect on fetal sexual development. This suggests the female structures normally develop from the paramesonephric ducts. In the male, the testes are thought to superimpose their effects onto this pattern so that female features are repressed.

When the paramesonephric ducts fuse, they bring two peritoneal folds into position (right and left broad ligaments) and two peritoneal pouches (rectouterine and vesicouterine pouches) are formed.

The mesonephric ducts and tubules regress in the female and only remnants may be found in the genital tract, i.e. the paraoophoron, appendix vesiculosa, duct of epoophoron and duct of Gartner.

Anomalies of the Uterine Tubes, Uterus and Vagina

Various abnormalities of the uterus result from abnormal fusion of the caudal portion of the paramesonephric ducts. Double uterus results from the failure of fusion of the inferior portion of the paramesonephric ducts. A single or double vagina may be associated with a double uterus. Bicornuate uterus is a doubling of the superior portion of the uterus. Failure of the duct(s) to develop also results in anomalies. The vaginal plate may fail to recanalise. The absence of a vagina and uterus are usually linked.

96. UTERINE TUBES, UTERUS AND VAGINA

STAGE 23

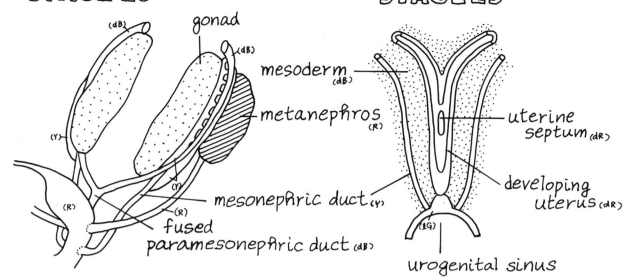

gonad

mesoderm (dB)

metanephros (R)

mesonephric duct (Y)

fused paramesonephric duct (dB)

(dB)

(dB)

(Y)

(R)

(R)

(Y)

STAGE 23

uterine septum (dR)

developing uterus (dR)

urogenital sinus

(lG)

WEEK 12

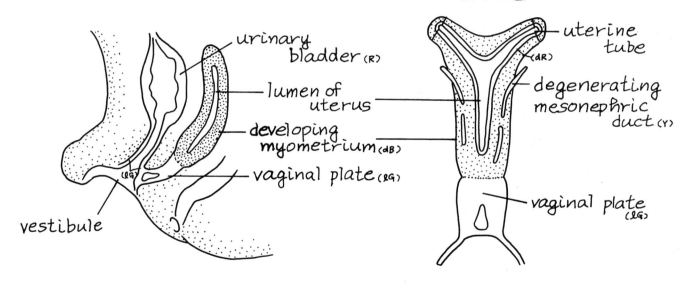

urinary bladder (R)

lumen of uterus

developing myometrium (dB)

vaginal plate (lG)

vestibule

(lG)

WEEK 12

uterine tube

(dR)

degenerating mesonephric duct (Y)

vaginal plate (lG)

6 MONTHS

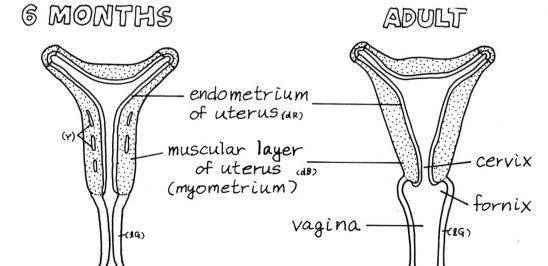

endometrium of uterus (dR)

muscular layer of uterus (dB) (myometrium)

(Y)

(lG)

hymen (lG)

ADULT

cervix

fornix

vagina

(lG)

97. Development of the Testes

As the primordial germ cells of male embryos reach the gonadal ridge on the posterior abdominal wall, prominent primary sex cords grow into the medulla. Here the cords form an anastomosis called the rete testis. The cords (now called seminiferous cords) are soon separat from the surface epithelium by a thick fibrous tunica albuginea. The seminiferous cords give rise to the rete testis, tubuli recti and seminiferous tubules. The seminiferous tubules are composed of two cell types: the spermatogonia derived from the primordial germ cells, and the sustentacular cells (of Sertoli). The Sertoli cells are derivatives of the surface epithelium.

The mesenchyme cells lying between the seminiferous tubules give rise to the interstitial cells (of Leydig). These cells produce testosterone and genital duct inducer and suppressor substances. Testosterone causes masculinisation of the external genitalia, while the inducer substances promote mesonephric duct development and the supressor substances inhibit paramesonephric duct development. The rete testis is connected to the mesonephric duct via 15–20 mesonephric tubules. Eventually the mesonephric tubules form the efferent ductules, while the duct forms the ductus epididymis.

97. DEVELOPMENT OF THE TESTES

STAGE 14

primordial germ cells (dR)

mesonephros
gonadal ridge (dB)

(dB)

(dB)

(R)

gut (R)

metanephric bud

STAGE 16 - 18

mesonephric
duct & tubule (dB)

developing
paramesonephric
duct (dR)

gonadal ridge (dB)

(QG)

(dB)

(dR)

(R)

primary sex cord (dB)

para-
mesonephric
duct (dR)

STAGE 20

(dB)

(dB)

(dB)

(R)

(dB)

(dR)

mesonephric duct

ureter

STAGE 20 - 23

tunica
albuginea (Y)

(dB)

(dR)

(R)

seminiferous
cord (dB)

surface epithelium (dB)

mesonephric
duct (dB)

paramesonephric
duct (dR)

WEEK 20

seminiferous tubule (dB)

septula testis (Y)

rete testis (dB)

(dB)

(dR)

ductus epididymis
(mesonephric duct) (dB)

degenerating
paramesonephric duct

(dB)

tunica
albuginea (Y)

ADULT

ductuli
efferentes
testis (B)

ductus
deferens (dG)

rete
testis (o)

tunica albuginea (Y)

ductus epididymis (dB)

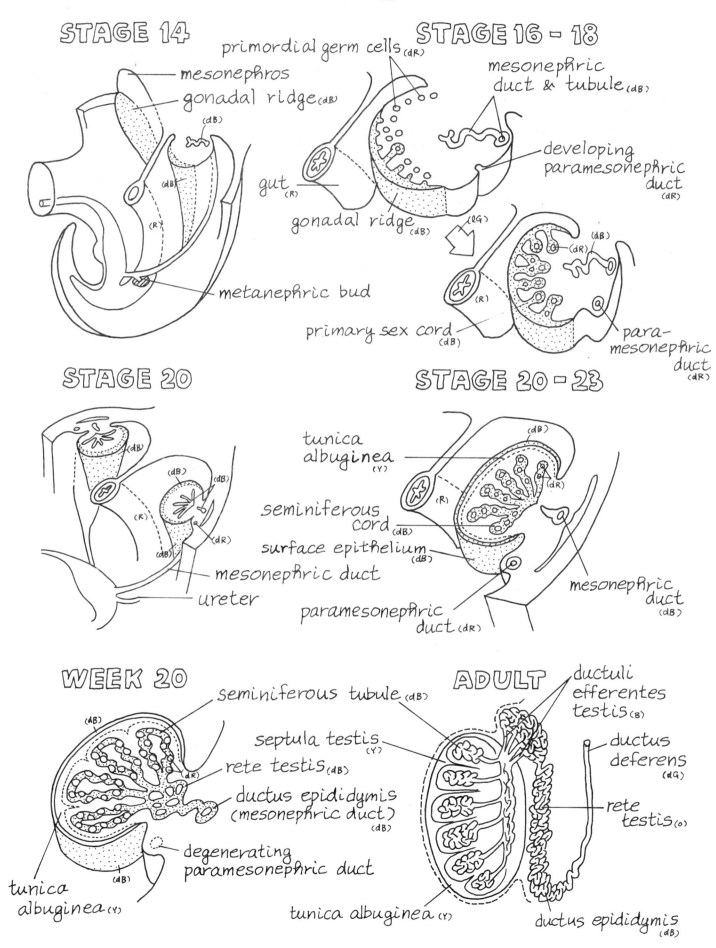

247

98. Early Female and Male Duct Systems

In the 'indifferent' stage, both male and female embryos have two pairs of ducts: mesonephric ducts and paramesonephric ducts.

The mesonephric ducts develop lateral to the mesonephric kidney. These will be retained in the male to form the highly convoluted epididymis, the ductus deferens and the ejaculatory duct. In the female, the mesonephric ducts largely disappear. A small part of the duct may be retained proximally as the appendix vesiculosa and distally as the duct of Gartner. This latter portion is equivalent to the portion which forms the ductus deferens and the ejaculatory duct in the male.

The paramesonephric ducts develop dorso-laterally to the mesonephric ducts. They form from mesodermal epithelium on the mesonephric kidney and enter the urogenital sinus. These ducts will be retained in the female to form the uterine tubes and uterovaginal primordium (see **96**. Uterine Tubes, Uterus and Vagina). In the male, the paramesonephric ducts largely disappear. When a small cranial part of the duct is retained, it is known as the appendix of the testis.

As the mesonephric kidney degenerates in the male, some tubules may persist as the paradidymis and the cranial end of the duct may persist as the appendix of the epididymis. In the female, tubules may be retained near the uterus as the paroophoron, and in the broad ligament as the epoophoron.

98. EARLY FEMALE AND MALE DUCT SYSTEMS

STAGE 16

STAGE 20

STAGE 23

WEEK 9 (FEMALE)

WEEK 9 (MALE)

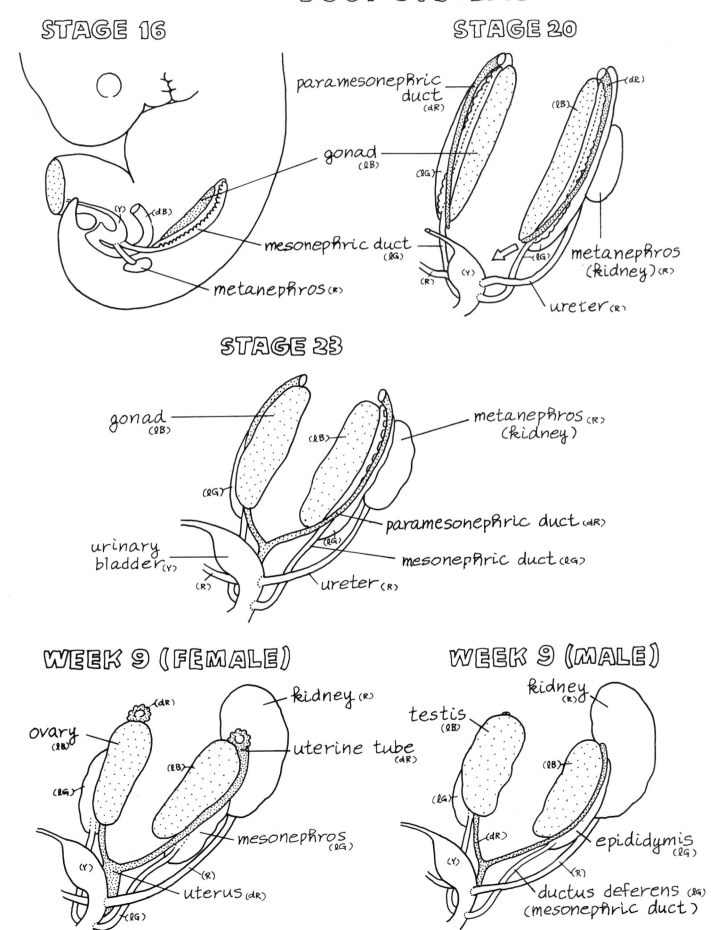

paramesonephric duct (dR)

gonad (lB)

mesonephric duct (lG)

metanephros (R)

metanephros (kidney) (R)

ureter (R)

gonad (lB)

metanephros (R) (kidney)

paramesonephric duct (dR)

urinary bladder (Y)

mesonephric duct (lG)

ureter (R)

kidney (R)

ovary (lB)

uterine tube (dR)

mesonephros (lG)

uterus (dR)

testis (lB)

kidney (R)

epididymis (lG)

ductus deferens (lG) (mesonephric duct)

99. External Genitalia: General

The external genitalia in both sexes are similar in the early stages of development. In the early embryo (Week 4, Stage 13), a genital tubercle develops at the cranial end of the cloacal membrane. Two pairs of folds or swellings appear on either side of this membrane and surround it; there is an inner urogenital fold, and an outer labioscrotal swelling. The genital tubercle in both sexes elongates to form a phallus.

The cloaca and cloacal membrane are divided by the urorectal septum in Week 6 into an urogenital sinus and urogenital membrane, and an anus and anal membrane. The two membranes rupture in Weeks 7–8 and form the urogenital orifice which continues onto the external surface of the phallus, and the anus.

Female or male characteristics develop between Weeks 9–12.

99. EXTERNAL GENITALIA : GENERAL

STAGE 13

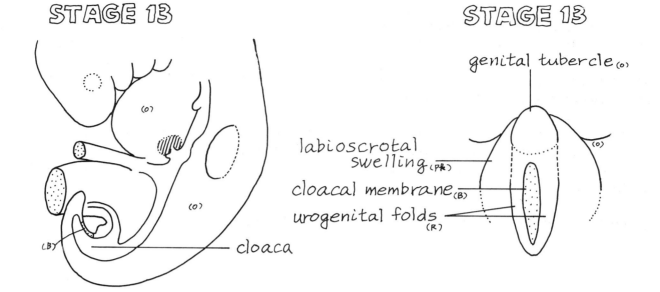

(O)

(O)

(O)

(B) — cloaca

STAGE 13

genital tubercle (O)

labioscrotal swelling (PR)

cloacal membrane (B)

urogenital folds (R)

(O)

STAGE 17

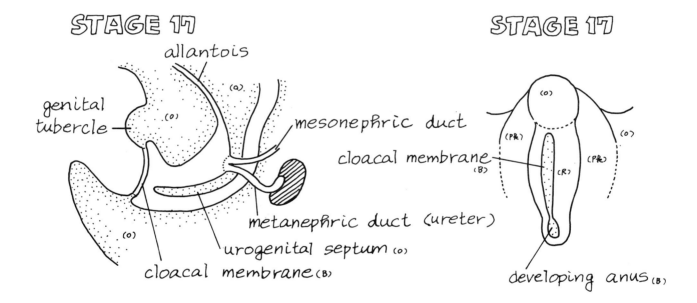

allantois

genital tubercle

(O)

(O)

(O)

mesonephric duct

cloacal membrane (B)

metanephric duct (ureter)

urogenital septum (O)

cloacal membrane (B)

STAGE 17

(O)

(PR)

(O)

cloacal membrane (B)

(R)

(PR)

developing anus (B)

WEEK 9

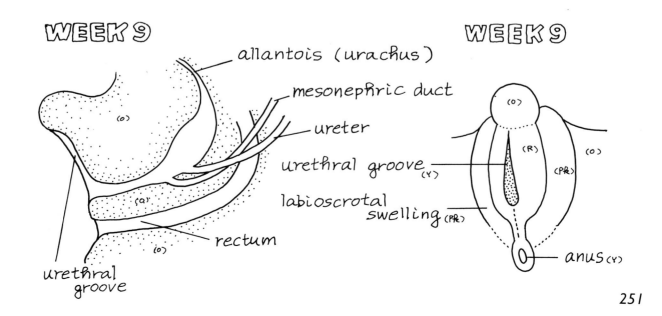

allantois (urachus)

mesonephric duct

ureter

urethral groove (Y)

labioscrotal swelling (PR)

rectum

urethral groove

(O)

(O)

(O)

WEEK 9

(O)

(R)

(O)

(PR)

anus (Y)

100. External Genitalia: Female

After the 'indifferent' stage, the external genitalia will develop and assume the characteristics of the female unless they are stimulated by the androgens which are secreted by the male fetus.

The relatively large 'indifferent' stage phallus becomes the clitoris in the female, and the urogenital membrane, which degenerates in Week 8, brings the urethral groove into continuity with the amniotic fluid. The urogenital folds then form the labia minora and fuse posteriorly at the frenulum. The labioscrotal swellings form the labia majora. They fuse anteriorly to form the mons pubis and anterior labial commissure, and fuse posteriorly to form the posterior labial commissure.

The cephalic portion of the urogenital sinus gives rise to the vestibule of the vagina. Opening into the vestibule are the vagina itself, the urethra, and the ducts of the greater vestibular glands. The hymen which is located across the vaginal lumen, usually ruptures during the perinatal period. This brings the lumen of the vagina into continuity with the vestibule. The hymen remains only as a thin membranous rim around the vaginal entrance.

Anomalies of the External Genitalia

Errors in development can result in an individual whose external genitalia are not in agreement with the morphology of their gonads. This condition is known as hermaphroditism.

100. EXTERNAL GENITALIA : FEMALE

WEEK 8

WEEK 11

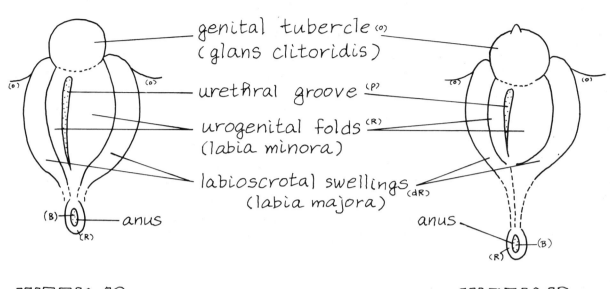

genital tubercle (O)
(glans clitoridis)

urethral groove (P)

urogenital folds (R)
(labia minora)

labioscrotal swellings (dR)
(labia majora)

anus

WEEK 12

WEEK 13

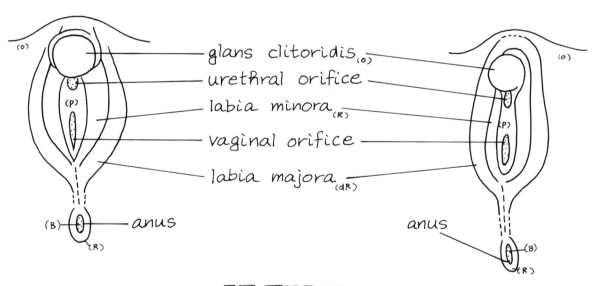

glans clitoridis (O)

urethral orifice

labia minora (R)

vaginal orifice

labia majora (dR)

anus

AT TERM

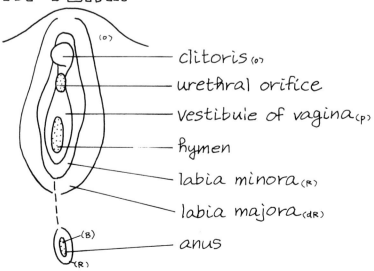

clitoris (O)

urethral orifice

vestibuie of vagina (P)

hymen

labia minora (R)

labia majora (dR)

anus

101. External Genitalia: Male

The male external genitalia differentiate when stimulated by androgens from the fetal testes.

The phallus elongates and forms the penis. As it grows, it brings the urogenital folds (on either side of the urogenital sinus) together in the midline. The folds form the lateral walls of the urethral groove. Endodermal cells lining the phallic portion of the urogenital sinus proliferate and form the urethral plate.

The urogenital folds fuse in the midline from proximal to distal to form the endodermal spongy urethra. The line of fusion of the urogenital folds is marked by the penile raphe. As fusion occurs the external urethral orifice moves towards the tip of the glans penis. The terminal portion of the urethra is ectodermal in origin. An ectodermal cord (glandular plate) grows towards and meets the spongy urethra.

The corpora cavernosa and corpus spongiosum are derived from mesenchyme in the phallus.

The labioscrotal swellings also fuse in the midline at a site marked by the scrotal raphe. They then form the scrotum.

The prepuce of the penis forms in Week 12, when a circular ectodermal ingrowth of a smaller diameter than the glans grows into the tip. This ingrowth will break down during infancy to allow the prepuce to retract.

Anomalies of the Male External Genitalia

Hypospadius results from the failure of fusion of the urogenital folds. The external urethral orifice is on the ventral surface of the body of the penis or the glans penis.

101. EXTERNAL GENITALIA: MALE

WEEK 8

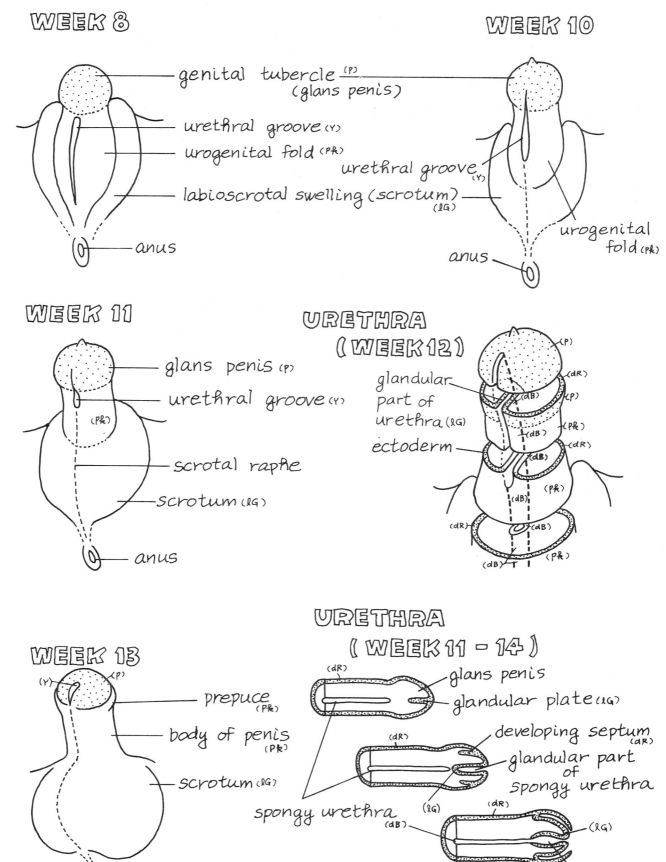

genital tubercle (P)
(glans penis)

urethral groove (Y)

urogenital fold (PK)

labioscrotal swelling (scrotum) (lG)

anus

WEEK 10

urethral groove (Y)

anus

urogenital fold (PK)

WEEK 11

glans penis (P)

urethral groove (Y)

(PK)

scrotal raphe

scrotum (lG)

anus

URETHRA (WEEK 12)

glandular part of urethra (lG)

ectoderm

(P)
(dR)
(dB)
(P)
(PK)
(dB)
(dR)
(dB)
(PK)
(dB)
(dR)
(dB)
(PK)
(dB) T

WEEK 13

(Y) (P)

prepuce (PK)

body of penis (PK)

scrotum (lG)

(lG)

URETHRA (WEEK 11 - 14)

(dR)

glans penis

glandular plate (lG)

developing septum (dR)

glandular part of spongy urethra

spongy urethra

(dR)

(lG)

(dB)

(lG)

prepuce (dR)

navicular fossa

102. Descent of the Ovaries

The ovaries are attached on their inferior pole to a ligament (gubernaculum) which forms from the degenerating mesonephros. This ligament extends through the developing anterior abdominal wall to attach to the internal aspect of the labioscrotal swelling.

A finger of abdominal peritoneum (processus vaginalis) follows the path of the gubernaculum and carries fascial layers of the abdominal wall before it. These layers then form the walls of the inguinal canal. In the female, the processus vaginalis normally disappears before birth.

In older fetuses, the gubernaculum is attached to the uterus near the entrance of the uterine tube. The cranial part of the gubernaculum forms the ovarian ligament while the caudal part forms the round ligament of the uterus. The round ligament then passes through the inguinal canal to end in the labium majus. The ovaries descend from the posterior abdominal wall to a position inferior to the pelvic brim and rotate so their caudal poles are directed medially. Their 'descent' is due to the relative movement as the cranial part of the abdomen grows away from the caudal part.

102. DESCENT OF THE OVARIES

STAGE 16

WEEK 9

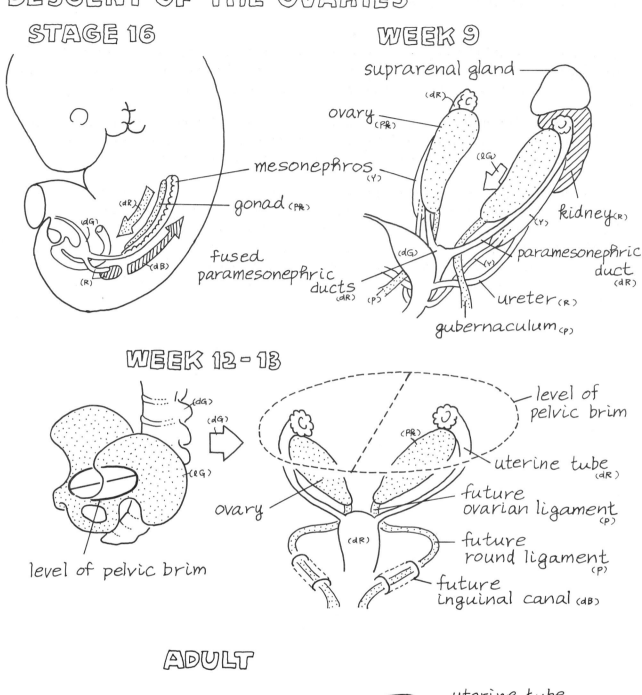

suprarenal gland

ovary (PK) (dR)

mesonephros (Y)

gonad (PK)

fused paramesonephric ducts (dR) (P)

kidney (R)

paramesonephric duct (dR)

ureter (R)

gubernaculum (P)

WEEK 12-13

(dG)

(dG)

(lG)

level of pelvic brim

level of pelvic brim

ovary

uterine tube (dR)

future ovarian ligament (P)

future round ligament (P)

future inguinal canal (dB)

(dR)

(PK)

ADULT

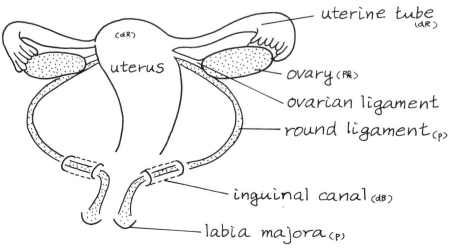

uterine tube (dR)

uterus (dR)

ovary (PK)

ovarian ligament

round ligament (P)

inguinal canal (dB)

labia majora (P)

257

103. Descent of the Testes

Inguinal canals develop in both sexes, but are only used in the male as a pathway for the descent of the testes from the posterior abdominal wall into the scrotum.

Each testis is attached on its inferior pole to a ligament (gubernaculum) which forms from the degenerating mesonephros. Both ligaments extend within the developing anterior abdominal walls to attach to the internal aspect of each labioscrotal swelling (future scrotum).

Ventral to each gubernaculum, an evagination of abdominal peritoneum (processus vaginalis) herniates along the path of the gubernaculum. Each processus carries with it and in front of it, extensions of certain layers of the abdominal wall. These extensions will form the walls of the inguinal canal. The deep inguinal ring forms where the processus pierces the internal aspect of the abdominal wall. Where the processus emerges through the abdominal wall, the superficial inguinal ring forms in the aponeurosis of the external oblique muscle.

The testes, their ductus deferens and vessels, 'descend' from the posterior abdominal wall as the trunk elongates. As they descend, they are encased in the fascial extensions of layers of the abdominal wall. They reach the deep inguinal ring by Week 28. This is largely a relative movement. Testicular movement through the inguinal canal and into the scrotum is external to the peritoneum and processus vaginalis. Movement through the canal is ill-understood. However, the gubernaculum appears to act as a guide-wire for each testis. It is believed that fetal androgens produced by the testis initiate and regulate testicular descent through the canal. The gubernaculum aids in anchoring the testis in the scrotum.

103. DESCENT OF THE TESTES

WEEK 9

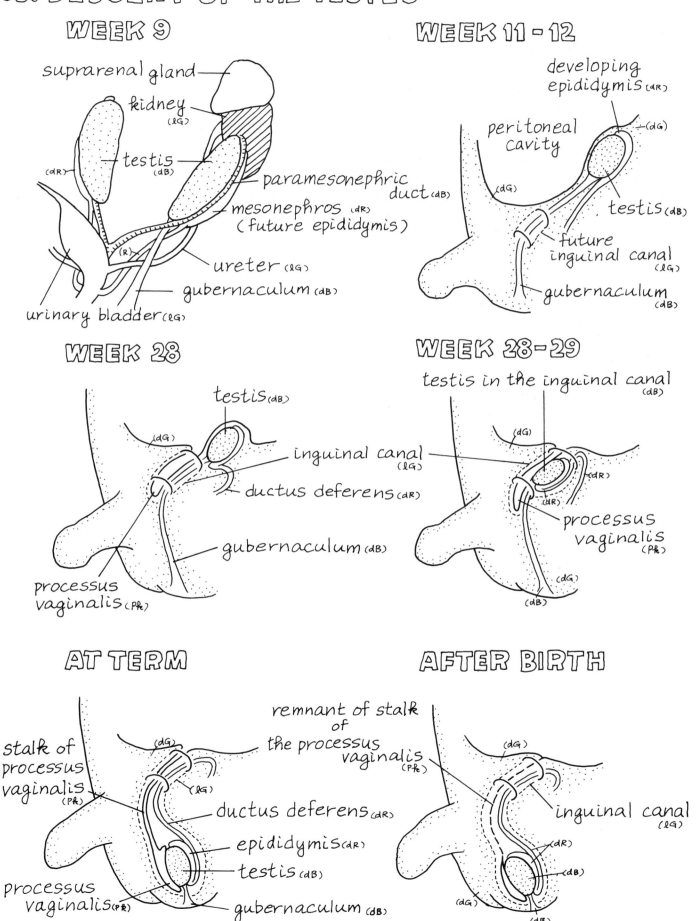

suprarenal gland

kidney (lG)

testis (dB)

(dR)

paramesonephric duct (dB)

mesonephros (dR) (future epididymis)

ureter (lG)

gubernaculum (dB)

urinary bladder (lG)

(R)

WEEK 11-12

developing epididymis (dR)

(dG)

peritoneal cavity

(dG)

testis (dB)

future inguinal canal (lG)

gubernaculum (dB)

WEEK 28

testis (dB)

(dG)

inguinal canal (lG)

ductus deferens (dR)

gubernaculum (dB)

processus vaginalis (PR)

WEEK 28-29

testis in the inguinal canal (dB)

(dG)

(dR)

(dR)

processus vaginalis (PR)

(dG)

(dB)

AT TERM

stalk of processus vaginalis (PR)

(dG)

(lG)

remnant of stalk of the processus vaginalis (PR)

ductus deferens (dR)

epididymis (dR)

testis (dB)

gubernaculum (dB)

processus vaginalis (PR)

AFTER BIRTH

(dG)

remnant of stalk of the processus vaginalis (PR)

inguinal canal (lG)

(dR)

(dB)

(dG)

(dB)

The testes begin to traverse the inguinal canal in Week 28 taking 2–3 days. By Week 32, the testes have entered the scrotum. They project into the distal end of the processus vaginalis. In the perinatal period, the connecting stalk of the processus vaginalis will degenerate leaving each testis surrounded by a peritoneal sac called the tunica vaginalis. The remnants of the gubernaculum remain as the gubernaculum testis.

In almost all (>97%) male full term neonates, the testes are located in the scrotum. Usually, in most of the remaining infants the testes will descend in the first 3 months. In some cases, testes remaining undescended will descend in response to androgenic hormones.

In the adult, certain layers of the embryonic abdominal wall covering the testes may easily be identified, i.e. the extension of the fetal transversalis fascia forms the adult internal spermatic fascia, the fetal internal oblique muscle forms the cremasteric muscle and fascia, and the fetal external oblique aponeurosis forms the external spermatic fascia.

Anomalies of Testicular Descent

Undescended testes (cryptorchidism) retained in or immediately outside the abdominal wall will not mature and causes sterility.

COVERINGS OF TESTIS

WEEK 11 - 12

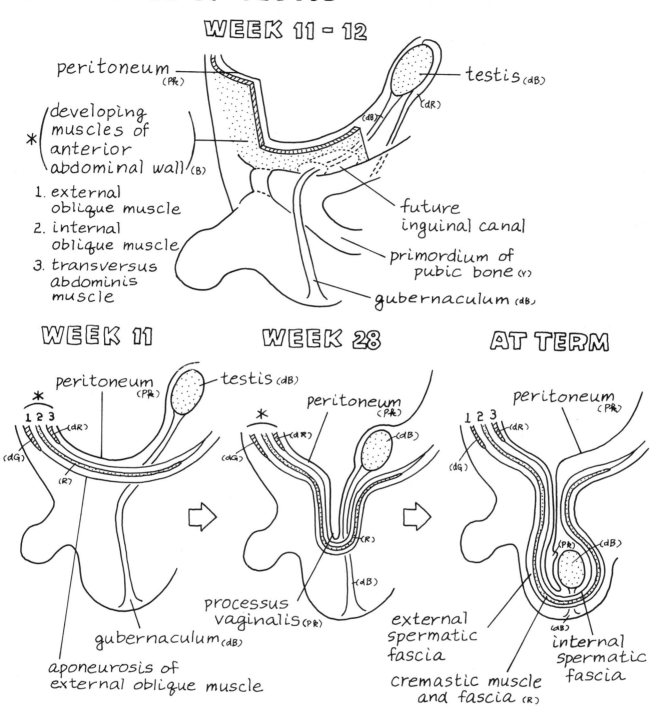

peritoneum _(PR)_

testis _(dB)_

_(dR)_

_(dB)_

* {
developing
muscles of
anterior
abdominal wall _(B)_
}

1. external
   oblique muscle
2. internal
   oblique muscle
3. transversus
   abdominis
   muscle

future
inguinal canal

primordium of
pubic bone _(Y)_

gubernaculum _(dB)_

WEEK 11

peritoneum _(PR)_

testis _(dB)_

*
1 2 3
_(dR)_
_(dG)_
_(R)_

gubernaculum _(dB)_

aponeurosis of
external oblique muscle

WEEK 28

peritoneum _(PR)_

*
_(dR)_
_(dG)_
_(dB)_

_(R)_

_(dB)_

processus
vaginalis _(PR)_

AT TERM

peritoneum _(PR)_

1 2 3
_(dR)_
_(dG)_

_(PR)_ _(dB)_

_(dB)_

external
spermatic
fascia

cremastic muscle
and fascia _(R)_

internal
spermatic
fascia

BONE DEVELOPMENT

104. Intramembranous Formation

Bones develop by either intramembranous or cartilaginous formation from mesenchymal cells which have condensed to form a model of the future bone.

In intramembranous bone formation, the mesenchymal model becomes highly vascularised and some cells differentiate to form osteoblasts (bone-forming cells). These specialised cells are widely separated, but remain in contact with each other by cellular processes. They deposit an osteoid tissue (pre-bone), and as this tissue is organised into bone, calcium phosphate is deposited. The calcium and phosphates required for ossification are supplied by the mother and are a heavy drain on the maternal system unless an adequate intake is in the diet.

As the bone forms, the osteoblasts become trapped. They are now known as osteocytes. Calcified matrix forms first in the centre of each island of uncalcified matrix. However, some osteoblasts remain around the perimeter of each island and continue to lay down new matrix.

As the bone becomes organised, spicules appear and coalesce to form lamellae. When lamellae form concentric layers around blood vessels, Haversian systems are developed.

Spiculated or spongy bone fills the core of the bone model while compact bone is laid down on the surface of the model. Bone marrow develops in the centre of the spongy bone from differentiating mesenchyme.

Bone is easily able to alter its shape during development. In addition to new bone being laid down by osteocytes, cells known as osteoclasts absorb bone. This allows the bones to be constantly remodelled in both the fetus and neonate.

Ossification begins in Week 6 and continues throughout the fetal period. The first bone to ossify is the clavicle.

BONE DEVELOPMENT
104. INTRAMEMBRANOUS FORMATION

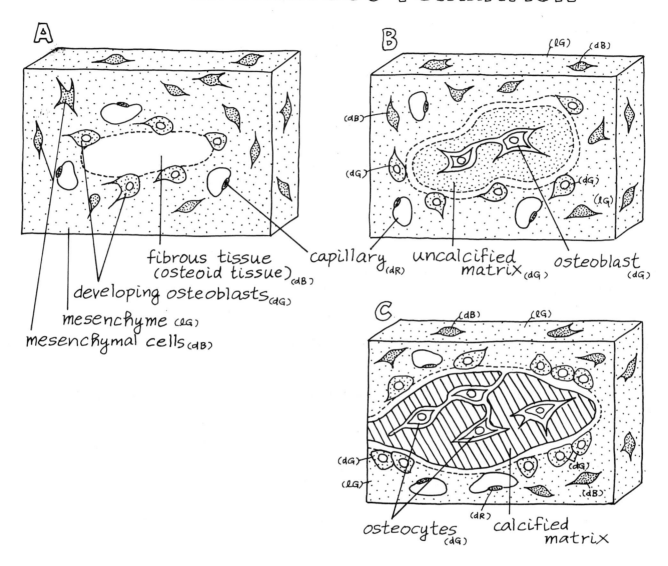

A

fibrous tissue (osteoid tissue)(dB)

capillary(dR)

developing osteoblasts(dG)

mesenchyme (ℓG)

mesenchymal cells(dB)

B

(ℓG) (dB)

(dB)

(dG) (dG)

(ℓG)

uncalcified matrix(dG)

osteoblast(dG)

C

(dB) (ℓG)

(dG)

(ℓG)

(dG)

(dB)

osteocytes(dG)

(dR) calcified matrix

105. Cartilage and Intracartilaginous Bone Formation

Cartilage

There are three types of cartilage: hyaline, elastic and fibrocartilage. All of these types form in a similar manner as the mesenchymal cells differentiate into chondroblasts. These cells then deposit matrix and collagen fibres so forming cartilage.

Intracartilaginous Bone Formation

Like intramembranous formation, intracartilaginous bone formation occurs in a model of the bone but in this case a cartilaginous model. A primary ossification centre appears in the cartilaginous model of the bone. This centre occurs in the shaft of the long bone which is called the diaphysis.

The periosteum of the bone forms from the perichondrium when a thin layer of bone is deposited under this layer. Then as the cartilage cells in the diaphysis enlarge, the matrix calcifies and the cells die. Arteries invade the diaphysis by first penetrating the periosteum, and then break up the arrangement of some of the cartilage cells into spicules. Some of this invading vascular connective tissue differentiates into haemopoietic cells so forming the bone marrow. Others differentiate into osteoblasts which deposit bone matrix onto the spicules of calcified cartilage.

The process of ossification continues towards the ends of the bone (epiphyses) at the diaphysio–epiphyseal junction. Lengthening of the bone occurs at the diaphysio–epiphyseal junction. Cartilage cells near the diaphysis divide and enlarge. The matrix calcifies, and becomes broken into spicules by the invading vascular connective tissue. Bone is deposited on these spicules. By birth the shafts of the bones are largely ossified, while the ends of epiphyses are still largely cartilaginous. Secondary ossification centres occur after birth in the epiphyses and ossification spreads throughout this area. The epiphyses are also invaded by vascular connective tissue. Only two areas at each end of a long bone remain cartilaginous; the articular cartilage and the epiphyseal cartilage plate separating the diaphysis and epiphysis.

The diameter of the bone is increased by bone deposition at the periosteal surface and by resorption at the medullary surface.

Remodelling of the bone is achieved by the balance of osteoblast and osteoclast activity. The relative amount of spongy bone and the bone marrow cavity are maintained by absorption of the bone on these spicules by the osteoclasts.

Irregular shaped bones develop similarly to the long bones. Ossification begins centrally and spreads peripherally in all directions.

Growth finally ceases at about age 20 years when the epiphyseal cartilage plate is replaced by spongy bone. The bone marrow cavities then become continuous between the diaphysis and the epiphyses.

105. CARTILAGE AND INTRACARTILAGINOUS BONE FORMATION

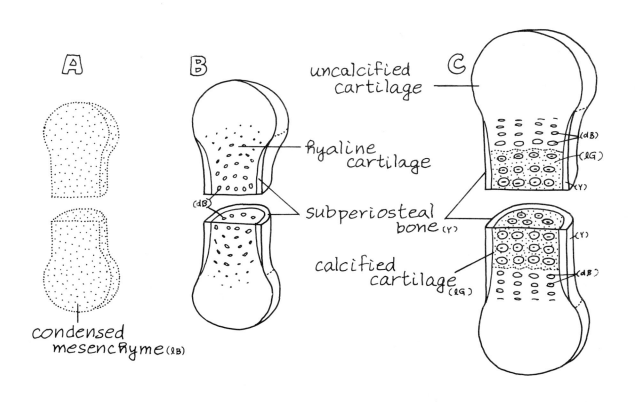

A

B

uncalcified
cartilage

C

hyaline
cartilage

(dB)

(ℓG)

(Y)

subperiosteal
bone (Y)

calcified
cartilage (ℓG)

(Y)

(dB)

(dB)

condensed
mesenchyme (ℓB)

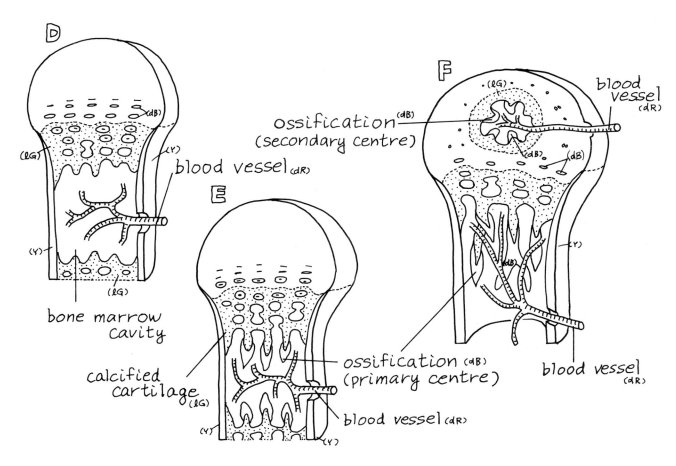

D

(dB)

(ℓG)

(Y)

blood vessel (dR)

(Y)

bone marrow
cavity

(ℓG)

F

(ℓG)

blood
vessel
(dR)

ossification (dB)
(secondary centre)

(dB)

(dB)

(Y)

E

calcified
cartilage
(ℓG)

(Y)

ossification (dB)
(primary centre)

blood vessel (dR)

blood vessel
(dR)

106. Skull

Neurocranium and Viscerocranium

The skull is divided into two main regions: the neurocranium or vault, and the viscerocranium or jaws.

Each of these regions has some membranous and some cartilaginous bones.

In general, the vault of the skull is membranous and the base of the skull cartilaginous in origin.

The bones form around the spinal cord, nerves, blood vessels etc., going to and from the brain and meninges. Some bones even form in several parts which ultimately fuse to form a single bone (e.g. occipital bone). The squamous temporal bone originates as a membranous part of the viscerocranium and later becomes part of the neurocranium.

The developing bones are separated from one another by fibrous tissue (sutures) which allows for the growth of the bone. As the brain increases in size, new bone is added to the outside surface of the bone and bone is removed from the inside surface.

There are several features which distinguish the fetal skull from the adult one. There are no developed paranasal sinuses, no erupted teeth, the lower margin of the orbit is level with the lower margin of the nose, there is a short external acoustic meatus and no mastoid process. These last two features are important in childbirth. The tympanic membrane is very near the surface and may be damaged during a forceps delivery. Due to the lack of the mastoid process, the facial nerve is exposed and may be injured.

106. SKULL
NEONATE

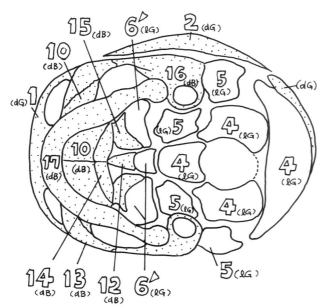

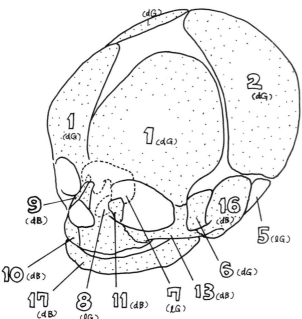

NEUROCRANIUM
▷ MEMBRANOUS
1 FRONTAL BONE (dG)
2 PARIETAL BONE (dG)
3 OCCIPITAL BONE (dG)
   (INTERPARIETAL PART)
6 PART OF SPHENOID (dG)

▷ CARTILAGINOUS
4 OCCIPITAL BONE (lG)
5 TEMPORAL BONE (lG)
   (PETROUS PART)
6' PART OF SPHENOID (lG)
7 ETHMOID (lG)
8 INFERIOR CONCHA (lG)

VISCEROCRANIUM
▷ MEMBRANOUS
9 NASAL BONE (dB)
10 MAXILLA (dB)
11 LACRIMAL BONE (dB)
12 VOMER (dB)
13 ZYGOMATIC BONE (dB)
14 PALATINE BONE (dB)
15 PTERYGOID PROCESS (dB)
16 TEMPORAL BONE (dB)
17 MANDIBULAR BONE (dB)
▷ CARTILAGINOUS
18 HYOID BONE (p)
19 STYLOID PROCESS (p)

Fontanelles

Large areas of fibrous tissue between the bones are called fontanelles. There are four major fontanelles: the anterior, the posterior, the sphenoidal and the mastoidal.

In childbirth, the fontanelles allow the bones of the skull vault to slide over each other. This moulding of the skull assists in the delivery of the head through the birth canal. Because the two frontal bones are fixed at the root of the nose, they are largely immobile. The shape of the skull vault returns to normal shortly after birth. In the neonate, the anterior fontanelle can be used clinically to assess dehydration or hydrocephalus. This fontanelle closes between 18–24 months, the anterolateral (sphenoidal) at 2–3 months, and the posterolateral (mastoidal) at 12 months. The two frontal bones fuse during year 2 and by year 8 the frontal or metopic suture is largely obliterated.

Anomalies of the Skull

Acrania or absence of the skull vault in association with anencephaly is incompatible with life.

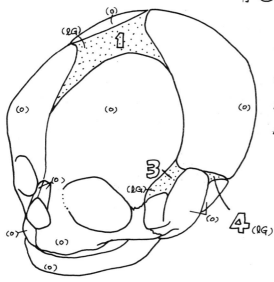

FONTANELLES

1 ANTERIOR FONTANELLE
2 POSTERIOR FONTANELLE
3 SPHENOIDAL FONTANELLE
4 MASTOIDAL FONTANELLE

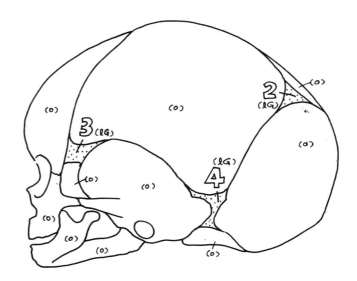

107. Vertebral Column

The sclerotome portion of each somite migrates into three general regions. One group migrates in the body wall, a second group migrates around the neural tube, and a third group migrates around the notochord.

The group migrating in the body wall will form the costal process of the vertebra. In the thoracic region, this group of cells will also form the ribs.

The group migrating around the neural tube will form the vertebral arch of the vertebra.

The group migrating around the notochord forms alternating regions cephalocaudally of loosely packed and densely packed groups of cells. Each sclerotome region, therefore, contributes a group of loosely packed cells and a group of densely packed cells opposite a myotome. Those densely packed cells immediately opposite the centre of each myotome form an intervertebral disc. The remaining densely packed cells fuse with the loosely packed cells lying immediately caudal and together form the centrum of the vertebra. This means each vertebra is formed from two different groups of sclerotome cells. Within each vertebra, the notochord degenerates; whilst within the embryonic intervertebral disc, the notochord expands to form the nucleus pulposus. Later, the anulus fibrosus forms around the nucleus pulposus and together they form the adult intervertebral disc.

107. VERTEBRAL COLUMN
STAGE 13

neural crest

sclerotome

(dB)

(ℓG)

(Y)

aorta
(R)

STAGE 13

caudal

(ℓG)

(dB)

(dB)

(R)

(ℓG)

(dB)

(R)

(R)

notochord
(Y)

aorta

(R)

intersegmental artery (R)

STAGE 16

notochord

spinal
ganglion

mesenchymal
primordia of
ribs and vertebrae (dB)

STAGE 16

(dB)

(ℓG)

(R)

(R)

(R)

spinal nerve

notochord (r)

STAGE 16

spinal nerve

notochord
(Y)

intersegmental
artery

sclerotomic
fissure

(dB)

(dB)

(dB)

A

chondrification
centre for
vertebral body (PR)

(R)

STAGE 17 - 18

neural
arch
(PR)

intersegmental
artery
(R)

A

(Y)

(PR)

(PR)

(dB)

(dB)

chondrification
centre
for rib
(PR)

B

intervertebral disc

(R)

A: segment derived from sclerotome   **B**: future vertebral body

Each mesenchymal vertebra develops chondrification centres and a cartilaginous model is formed. Ossification begins at the end of the embryonic period and continues until age 25 years. Three primary centres of ossification occur in each vertebra and by birth the vertebrae are each composed of three bones separated by cartilage. Secondary ossification centres appear after puberty and ossification is completed at 25 years.

The intersegmental arteries become the intercostal arteries and come to lie on either side of each vertebral body. The spinal nerves emerge between the mesenchymal vertebrae.

Anomalies of the Vertebral Column

Vertebra

In spina bifida occulta the neural arch fails to fuse and remains as two halves.

Notochord

Chordoma is a neoplasm of a persisting remnant of the notochord.

Note: The development of the vertebral column is controversial (see Johnson, D. R., 'The Genetics of the Skeleton').

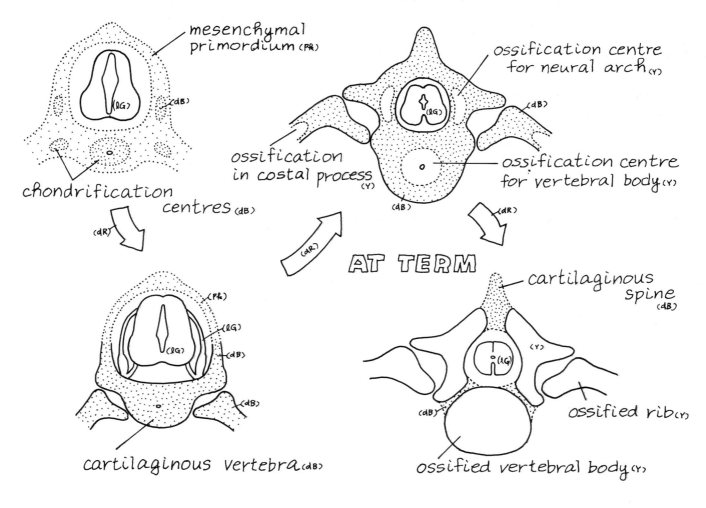

STAGE 17 - 20

mesenchymal
primordium (PR)

(ℓG)

(dB)

chondrification
centres (dB)

(dR)

(PR)

(ℓG)

(ℓG)

(dB)

(dB)

(dB)

cartilaginous vertebra (dB)

WEEK 9 - 10

ossification centre
for neural arch (Y)

(ℓG)

(dB)

ossification
in costal process
(Y)

ossification centre
for vertebral body (Y)

(dB)

(dR)

(dR)

AT TERM

cartilaginous
spine
(dB)

(Y)

(ℓG)

(dB)

ossified rib (Y)

ossified vertebral body (Y)

108. Appendicular Skeleton and Joints

The appendicular skeleton consists of the limb bones and pectoral and pelvic girdles. The pectoral girdle and arms appear before the pelvic girdle and legs; their mesenchymal models initially appear in Week 5. By Week 6, they have differentiated into hyaline cartilage models and by Week 8 enchondral ossification begins in the long bones. All the primary ossification centres are present at Weeks 7–12. These centres occur towards the middle of the bone and are referred to as the diaphysis. Although some secondary centres of ossification occur before birth, most appear after birth. Bone ossified from these centres is referred to as the epiphysis.

The first bone in the appendicular skeleton to ossify (Week 6) is the clavicle (membranous formation). Later, cartilage develops at both ends.

By ultrasound scans, it is possible to determine the length of the femur and diagnose achondroplasia and other conditions of the bone.

Anomalies of the Appendicular Skeleton

Defects in the epiphyseal cartilage plates during enchondral ossification cause a form of dwarfism known as achondroplasia.

Agenesis of the thyroid gland or a deficiency of fetal thyroid hormone results in cretinism. This is characterised by mental deficiency, neurological and auditory disorders and skeletal abnormalities.

Development of Joints

There are three main types of joints: fibrous, cartilaginous and synovial. As two adjacent bones develop, they are separated from one another by interzonal mesenchyme. In a fibrous joint, the interzonal mesenchyme becomes fibrous connective tissue, whilst in a cartilaginous joint, the interzonal mesenchyme becomes fibrocartilage or hyaline cartilage.

During development of a synovial joint, the peripheral interzonal mesenchyme differentiates into the capsule and ligaments. The mesenchyme disappears centrally leaving the joint cavity and where it lines the capsule forms the synovial membrane lining the capsule and articular surfaces.

108. APPENDICULAR SKELETON AND JOINTS
STAGE 18   WEEK 9-10

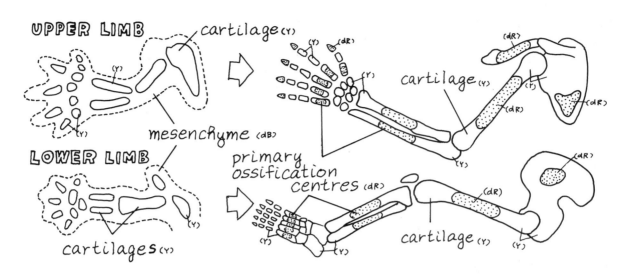

OSSIFICATION AT BIRTH

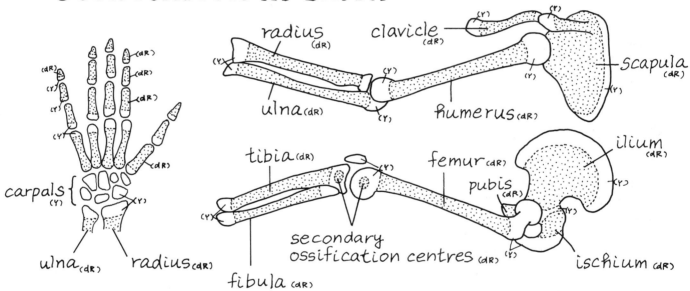

DEVELOPMENT OF A JOINT

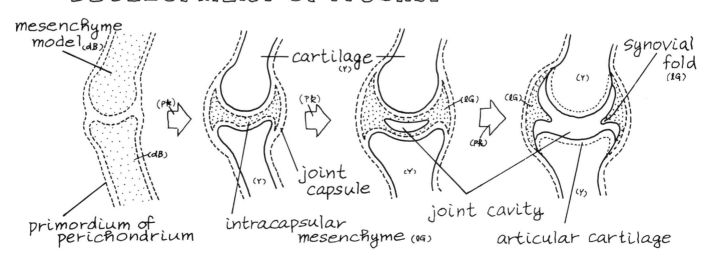

MUSCLES

109. General

Most skeletal, smooth and cardiac muscles develop from the mesoderm layer (see **13**. Derivatives of the Germ Layers: Ectoderm, Mesoderm and Endoderm). There are exceptions, however, e.g. the neural crest contributes to head mesenchyme which subsequently develops into muscles.

The mesenchyme cells differentiate to form muscle precursor cells called myoblasts. The different muscle types are described in **110–112**.

Anomalies of Muscle Formation

Muscle variation is very common and is often of little functional importance. Certain muscles may also be missing on one side or on both sides of the body.

MUSCLES

109. GENERAL

▷ MUSCLES OF THE HEAD AND NECK

▷ BRANCHIAL ARCHES (dB)
ARCH 1 : MUSCLES OF MASTICATION
ARCH 2 : FACIAL MUSCLES
ARCH 3 : STYLOPHARYNGEUS
ARCH 4 & 6 : PHARYNGOLARYNGEAL
(STERNOCLEIDOMASTOID, TRAPEZIUS)
▷ PREOTIC MYOTOMES (dG)
OCCULAR MUSCLES
▷ OCCIPITAL MYOTOMES
TONGUE MUSCLES (Y)

▷ OTHER MUSCLES

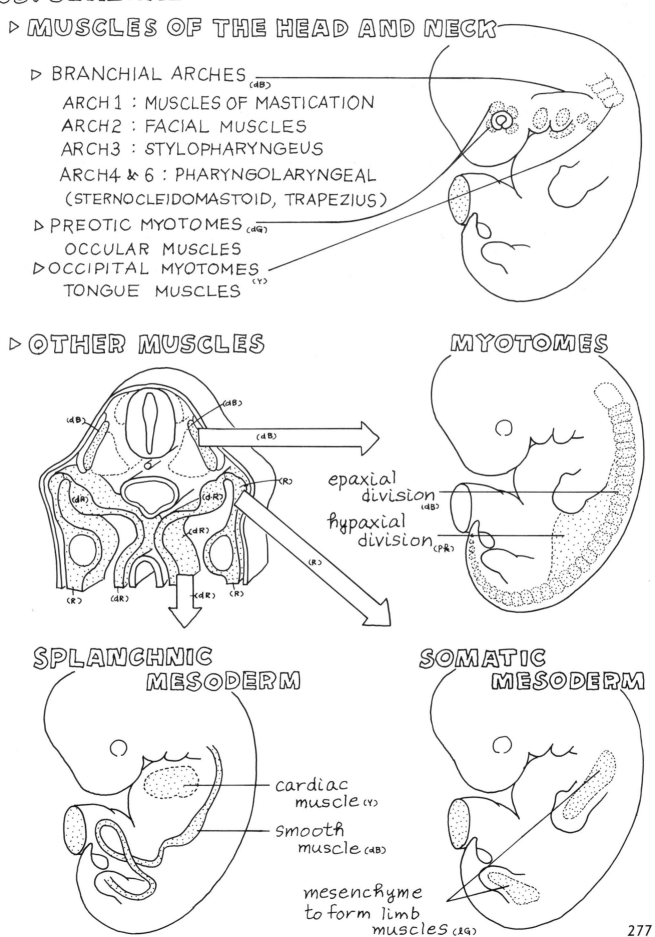

MYOTOMES

epaxial division (dB)
hypaxial division (PR)

SPLANCHNIC MESODERM

cardiac muscle (Y)
smooth muscle (dB)

SOMATIC MESODERM

mesenchyme to form limb muscles (lG)

277

110. Skeletal

As the myoblasts differentiate to form skeletal muscle, they develop elongated cell bodies and nuclei. Several cells then fuse together to form a multinucleated myotube whose cytoplasm contains myofilaments. Myofibrils differentiate in the cytoplasm and the long myotube cells become known as muscle fibres. These fibres or groups of fibres have an external lamina which establishes their perimeter.

Mesenchyme which develops into skeletal muscle has various origins. The limb musculature forms *in situ* from somatic mesenchyme, while most trunk muscles develop from mesenchyme which migrates from the myotome region of the somites. In the head, mesenchyme migrating from the branchial arches forms many face, jaw, neck and shoulder muscles. The tongue muscles, however, differentiate from three indistinct occipital myotomes supplied by the hypoglossal nerve (XII).

The skeletal muscles of the trunk are derived from two subdivisions of the myotome region of the somites. The small dorsal epaxial division develops into the extensor muscles of the neck, vertebral column and lumbar musculature. This division is supplied by the dorsal primary ramus of the spinal nerve. The large ventral hypaxial division develops into the scalene, prevertebral, geniohyoid and infrahyoid muscles, the lateral and ventral flexors of the vertebral column, quadratus lumborum, muscles of the pelvic diaphragm and probably those of the sex organs and anus. This division is supplied by the ventral primary ramus of the spinal nerve.

Movements of the limbs are detected by ultrasound scans from Week 7. The fetus is normally very active and it moves both arms and legs to adjust and change its position *in utero.*

110. SKELETAL

STAGE 12

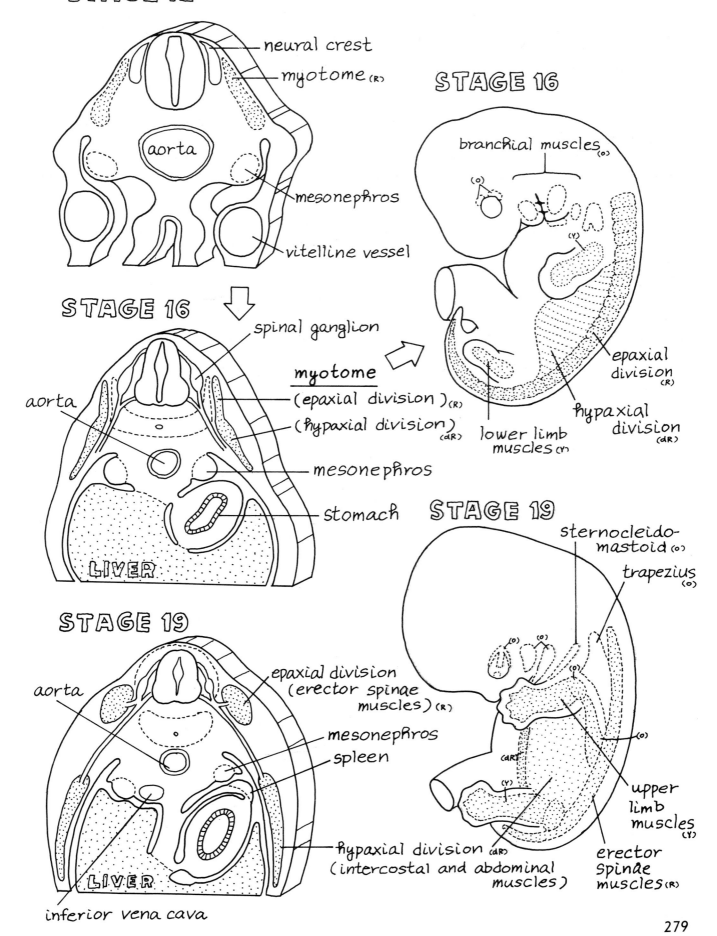

neural crest

myotome (R)

aorta

mesonephros

vitelline vessel

STAGE 16

branchial muscles (o)

(o)

(Y)

epaxial division (R)

lower limb muscles (Y)

hypaxial division (dR)

STAGE 16

spinal ganglion

aorta

myotome

(epaxial division) (R)

(hypaxial division) (dR)

mesonephros

stomach

LIVER

STAGE 19

sternocleido-mastoid (o)

trapezius (o)

(o) (o)

(o)

(dR)

(Y)

(o)

upper limb muscles (Y)

erector spinae muscles (R)

STAGE 19

aorta

epaxial division (erector spinae muscles) (R)

mesonephros

spleen

LIVER

hypaxial division (dR) (intercostal and abdominal muscles)

inferior vena cava

111. Smooth

Myoblasts which will form smooth muscle usually differentiate from mesenchyme. They are identifiable by their elongated nuclei, contractile elements and an external lamina. The developing muscle fibres form bundles or sheets.

Smooth muscles develop from several different types of mesenchyme. The smooth muscle of the gut forms from the surrounding splanchnic mesenchyme as it condenses around the endodermal gut. However, blood vessel wall smooth muscle also forms from somatic mesenchyme. Some other smooth muscles develop from mesenchyme derived from ectoderm (e.g. the iris muscles).

111. SMOOTH

ORIGINS OF SMOOTH MUSCLES

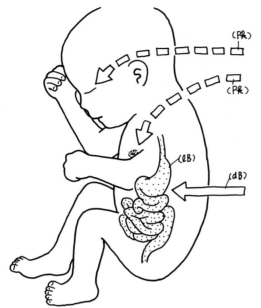

ECTODERM

sphincter and dilator pupillae

myoepithelial cells

(sweat and mammary gland)

MESODERM

smooth muscles surrounding
the primitive gut and its derivatives

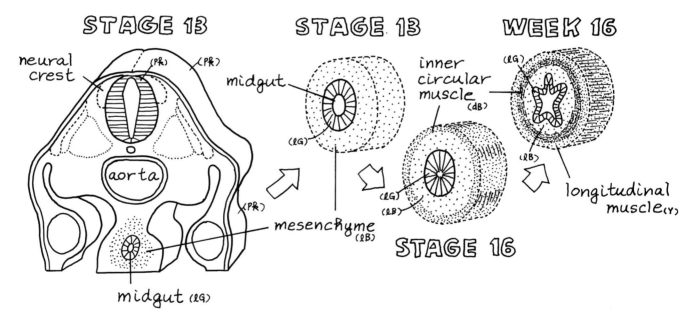

STAGE 13   **STAGE 13**   **WEEK 16**

neural crest

(PR)   (PR)

midgut

inner circular muscle (dB)

(lG)

aorta

(lG)

(PR)

mesenchyme (lB)

(lG)
(lB)

longitudinal muscle (Y)

STAGE 16

midgut (lG)

112. Cardiac

The early, single heart tube is surrounded by a layer of splanchnic mesenchyme. When this condenses it forms a myoepicardial mantle around the heart tube. This will give rise to the muscle layer of the heart (myocardium) and the visceral pericardium or epicardium. The mantle and tube are separated by a gelatinous layer of cardiac jelly. During Week 4, cardiac muscle develops in this mantle from single, differentiating cells which group together and adhere. Intercalated discs arise between the adhering cells.

The heart begins to beat between Weeks 3–4 and its muscles are well developed by birth.

112. CARDIAC

STAGE 9

plane of the section

AMNIOTIC CAVITY

heart tube

pericardial cavity

YOLK SAC

splanchnic mesoderm (dB) (myoepicardium)

STAGE 9

dorsal aorta   neural groove

(dB)

(Y)

FOREGUT

(dB)

(Y)

(Y)

(dB)

endocardium (P)   fusing heart tubes   cardiac jelly (Pk)

STAGE 10

neural tube

(Y)

(Y)

(Pk)

endo-cardium (P)

myoepicardial mantle (dB)

STAGE 10 - 13

(Pk)

myo-epicardial mantle (dB)

cardiac jelly

(P)

(dB)

epicardium (dB)

myocardium (lB)

STAGE 11 - 12

epicardium (dB)

developing myocardium (lB)

cardiac jelly (Pk)

endocardium (P)

endocardium (P)

ADULT

cardiac muscle (lB)

LIMBS

113. Formation and Rotation of Limbs

Limb Buds

The limb buds appear late in Week 4. The upper limb bud is found opposite spinal levels C5–T1 by Days 26–27, and the lower limb bud opposite L2–S3 by Day 28. Much later, during Weeks 6–8, the limbs will descend to their normal positions relative to the trunk. Each limb bud is composed of a core of somatic mesoderm covered by a glove of ectoderm. The mesenchyme will contribute to the bones, joints, muscles and dermis, and the ectoderm to the skin, nails, hair, sebaceous and sweat glands. At the tip of the bud a thickening, the apical ectoderm ridge, exerts an inductive influence on the growth and proliferation of the limb mesenchyme. The thumb (or big toe) denotes the preaxial border and the little finger (or toe) denotes the postaxial border.

The early stages of limb development are similar in both the upper and lower limbs. However, the upper limb development precedes the lower limb because of its more cranial position and its more highly oxygenated blood supply.

Muscles

The muscles form primarily from mesenchyme *in situ*. This musculature generally is divided into dorsal (extensor) and ventral (flexor) groups.

Hand and Foot Plate

During Week 5, a paddle-shaped hand or foot plate forms at the distal end of each limb bud. During Week 6, their mesenchyme condenses to form one digital ray for each future digit of the hand and a similar process occurs in the foot plate in Week 7. Notches appear and programmed cell death occurs between the digital rays to separate the individual digits in Week 8.

Limb Rotation

The upper and lower limb buds originally project at an angle of 90° from the body wall. The upper limb, while developing an elbow, rotates so that the hands come to lie over the thorax and the elbow points posteriorly. The future knee region comes to face anteriorly with the flexors lying posteriorly and the extensors anteriorly.

LIMBS

113. FORMATION AND ROTATION OF LIMBS

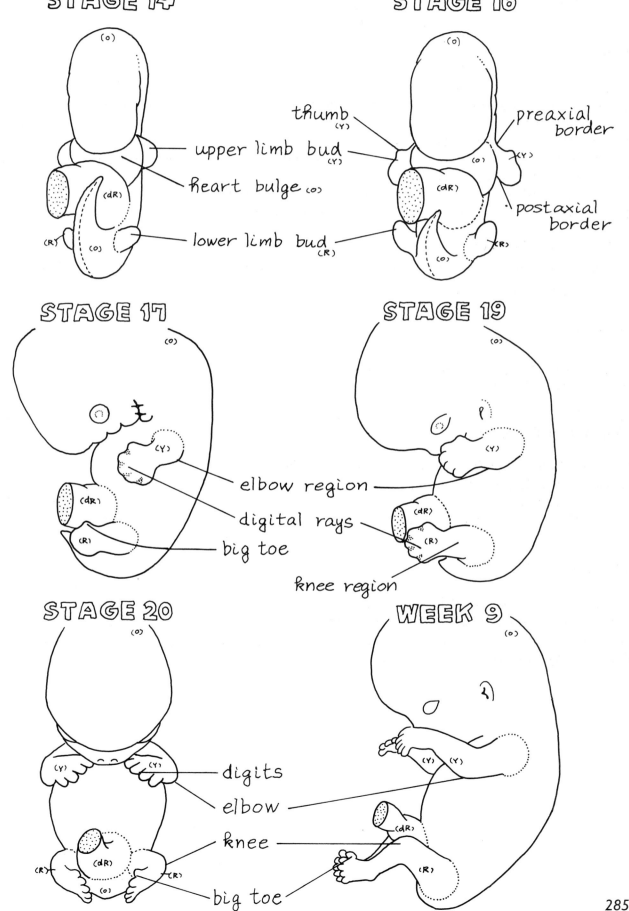

STAGE 14

(o)

upper limb bud

heart bulge (o)

(dR)

(R)

lower limb bud (R)

(o)

STAGE 16

(o)

thumb (Y)

(Y)

preaxial border

(o) (Y)

(dR)

postaxial border

(o)

(R)

STAGE 17

(o)

(Y)

elbow region

(dR)

digital rays

(R)

big toe

STAGE 19

(o)

(Y)

(dR)

(R)

knee region

STAGE 20

(o)

(Y) (Y)

digits

elbow

(dR)

knee

(R) (R)

(o)

big toe

WEEK 9

(o)

(Y) (Y)

(dR)

(R)

114. Skeleton and Innervation of Limbs

Bones, Joints and Nerves

The limbs elongate by proliferation of their mesenchyme. The bones form first as mesenchymal models in Week 5. Centres of chondrification appear in this week and by Week 6 the entire skeleton of the limbs is cartilaginous. Primary ossification centres appear in the middle of the long bones in Week 7.

The ventral rami of the spinal nerves, C5–T1 and L2–S3, invade the upper and lower limb buds respectively.

The cutaneous branches of the main nerves of the limb each supply an area of skin (dermatome) which is arranged segmentally on the limb bud. As the limbs grow and rotate, the dermatomes adjust to form the adult pattern of innervation.

Anomalies of the Limbs

Clubfoot is a common deformity involving the talus. Abnormal positioning of the feet *in utero* may be a contributing factor.

Congenital dislocation of the hips is a common deformity attributed to general laxity of the joint and underdevelopment of the acetabulum.

114. SKELETON AND INNERVATION OF LIMBS

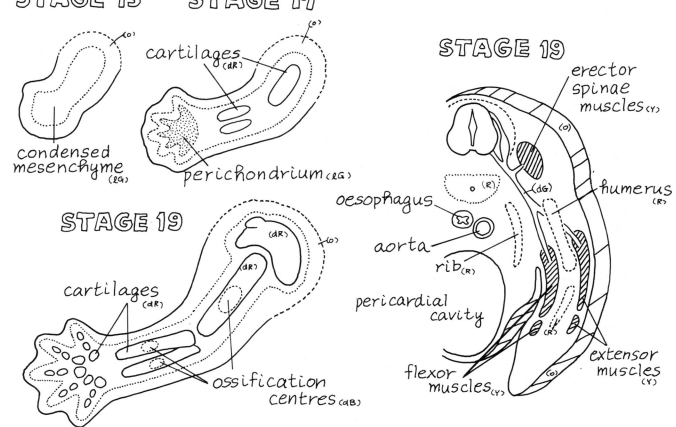

STAGE 15   STAGE 17

cartilages (dR)

condensed mesenchyme (lG)

perichondrium (lG)

STAGE 19

STAGE 19

cartilages (dR)

ossification centres (dB)

erector spinae muscles (Y)

oesophagus

aorta

rib (R)

pericardial cavity

humerus (R)

flexor muscles (Y)

extensor muscles (Y)

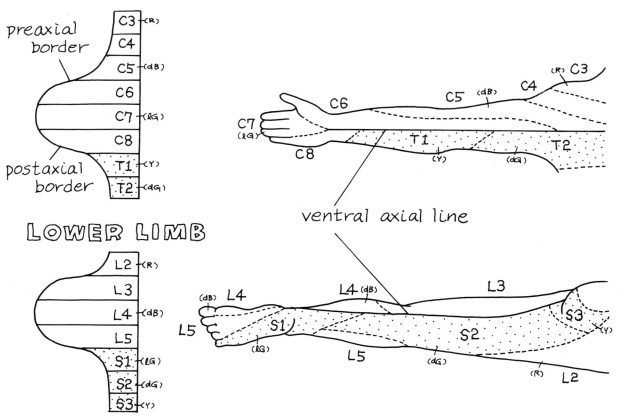

UPPER LIMB

preaxial border

postaxial border

C3	(R)
C4	
C5	(dB)
C6	
C7	(lG)
C8	
T1	(Y)
T2	(dG)

C6
C5 (dB)
C4
C3 (R)
C7 (lG)
C8
T1 (Y)
T2 (dG)

ventral axial line

LOWER LIMB

L2	(R)
L3	
L4	(dB)
L5	
S1	(lG)
S2	(dG)
S3	(Y)

L4 (dB)
L4 (dB)
L3
L5
S1
S2
S3 (Y)
L5 (dG)
L2 (R)

INTEGUMENTARY SYSTEM

115. Skin

The epidermis is an ectodermal derivative, while the dermis is mesodermal in origin. The melanocytes are neural crest derivatives which migrate to the dermo-epithelial junction.

The early epidermis is composed of a single layer of cells which proliferates to form an external squamous epithelium known as periderm. This external layer undergoes continual keratinisation and desquamation while being replaced by the underlying basal layer. The desquamated cells contribute to the vernix caseosa, a white cheesy protective coat on the fetal skin. Other components of the vernix caseosa are hair, sebum and amniotic cells.

As the basal layer (stratum germinativum) continues to proliferate, an intermediate layer forms which will later form the stratum corneum, stratum lucidum, stratum granulosum and stratum spinosum. The stratum germinativum continues to proliferate and downgrowths (epidermal ridges) extend into the dermis below. All the layers of epidermis found in the adult are present at birth.

The dermis is primarily derived from the somatic mesoderm with a contribution from the dermatomes of the somites. The mesenchyme differentiates into elastic and collagenous connective tissue. When the epidermal ridges form, dermal papillae project into the epidermis. Fingerprints appear between Weeks 13–16.

Blood vessels and sensory nerves develop in relation to the dermal papillae.

Anomalies of the Skin

Angiomas are benign endothelial cell tumours containing blood. Hemangiomas (e.g. port wine stain) are common infant vascular malformations.

INTEGUMENTARY SYSTEM

115. SKIN

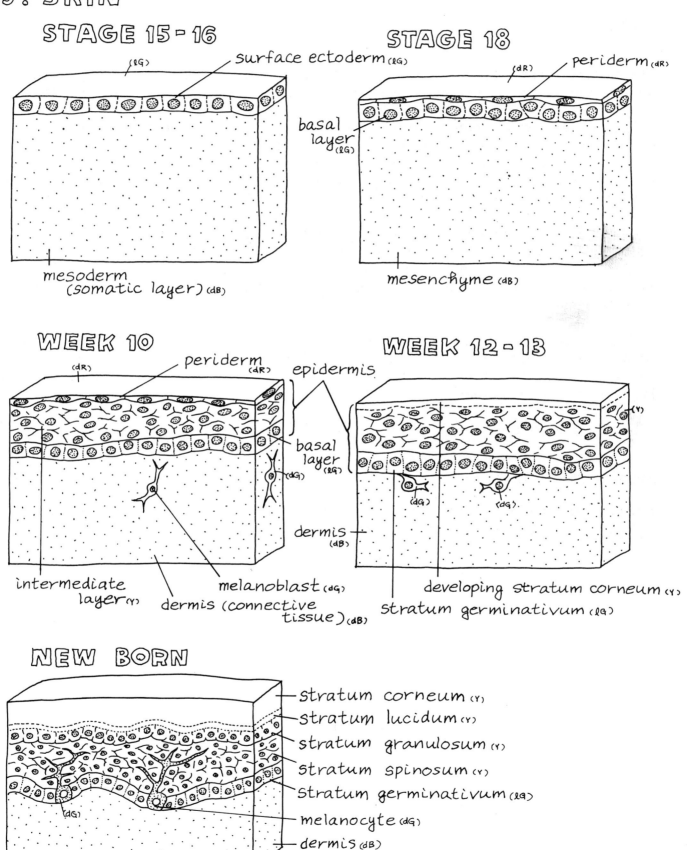

STAGE 15-16

(ℓG)

surface ectoderm (ℓG)

mesoderm
(somatic layer) (dB)

STAGE 18

(dR)

periderm (dR)

basal layer (ℓG)

mesenchyme (dB)

WEEK 10

(dR)

periderm (dR)

epidermis

basal layer (ℓG)

(dG)

intermediate layer (Y)

melanoblast (dG)

dermis (connective tissue) (dB)

WEEK 12-13

(Y)

(dG)

(dG)

dermis (dB)

developing stratum corneum (Y)

stratum germinativum (ℓG)

NEW BORN

stratum corneum (Y)

stratum lucidum (Y)

stratum granulosum (Y)

stratum spinosum (Y)

stratum germinativum (ℓG)

melanocyte (dG)

dermis (dB)

(dG)

116. Hair and Skin Glands

Hair

Hair follicles develop when a layer of the epidermis (stratum germinativum) proliferates and downgrowths penetrate the dermis. The deepest part of the follicle forms a hair bulb whose epithelial cells create a germinal matrix. This will give rise to the hair and the walls of the downgrowth will form the epithelial root sheath. Mesenchyme deep to the hair bulb invaginates to become a hair papilla, while those cells surrounding the epithelial root sheath condense to form the dermal root sheath. A hair is produced when cells in the germinal matrix proliferate and become the hair shaft which becomes keratinised as it elongates.

The primary hairs are evident in the chin, upper lip and eyebrows in the early fetal period (Weeks 9–12). These fine hairs are called lanugo and eventually cover most of the fetal skin (Month 7). They are continually shed and contribute to the white, waxy vernix caseosa covering and protecting the skin. Most of these hairs are shed around birth. Fine 'down' hairs replace these primary hairs.

Mesenchyme adjacent to the hair follicle differentiates to form arrector pili muscle. Melanoblasts (neural crest derivatives) migrate into the hair bulb and differentiate into melanocytes. These cells produce melanin which determines hair colour.

Sebaceous Glands

Sebaceous glands develop as outgrowths on the side of the hair follicle (Month 4). These glandular buds branch repeatedly to form a system of solid ducts and alveoli. The ducts canalise when the central cells break down and are extruded into the hair follicles and onto the skin. The oily secretion of the sebaceous glands (sebum) is a major constituent of the vernix caseosa.

Sweat Glands

Large sweat glands are associated with hairs and open into the hair follicle. They develop from the stratum germinativum which also gives rise to the hair itself. The large sweat glands are primarily limited to the axilla, areolae of the breasts and pubic region.

Other sweat glands open directly onto the skin surface and they develop as downgrowths of the epidermal layer into the dermis. As the solid bud grows, its distal end coils and differentiates to form the secretory part of the sweat gland. The peripheral cells differentiate to form secretory and myoepithelial cells while the central cells degenerate as the gland canalises.

Anomalies Associated with the Hair and Skin Glands

Albinos lack melanin and as a result have white hair.

116. HAIR AND SKIN GLANDS

HAIR, SEBACEOUS GLANDS

WEEK 12

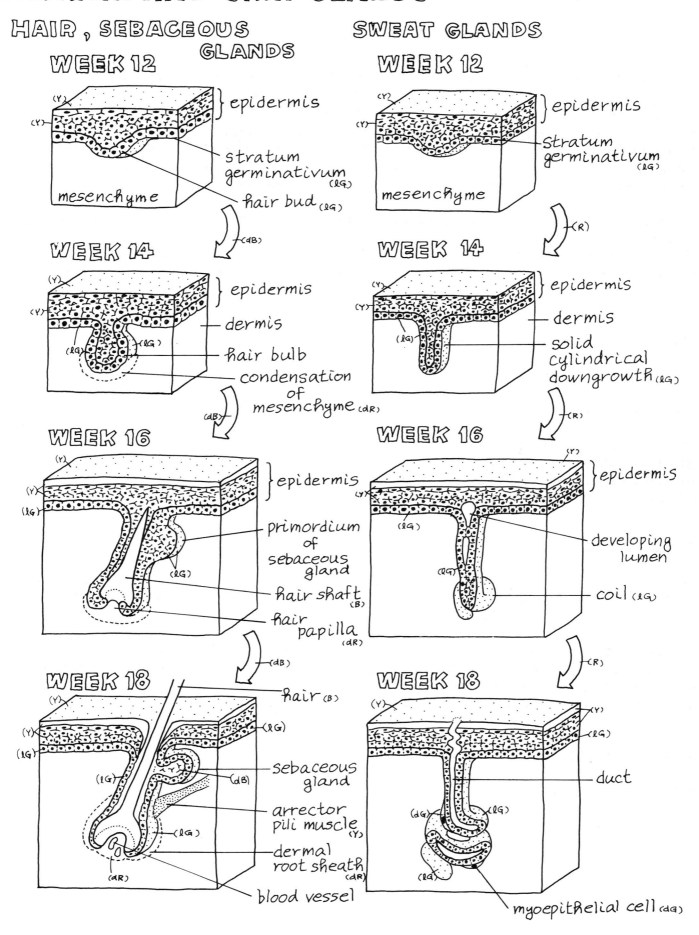

epidermis

stratum germinativum (lG)

mesenchyme

hair bud (lG)

WEEK 14

epidermis

dermis

hair bulb

condensation of mesenchyme (dR)

WEEK 16

epidermis

primordium of sebaceous gland

hair shaft (B)

hair papilla (dR)

WEEK 18

hair (B)

sebaceous gland

arrector pili muscle (Y)

dermal root sheath (dR)

blood vessel

SWEAT GLANDS

WEEK 12

epidermis

stratum germinativum (lG)

mesenchyme

WEEK 14

epidermis

dermis

solid cylindrical downgrowth (lG)

WEEK 16

epidermis

developing lumen

coil (lG)

WEEK 18

duct

myoepithelial cell (dG)

117. Nails

The nail fields of both the fingers and the toes first appear at Week 10 as ectodermal thickenings on the tips of each digit. They then acquire a nerve supply from the ventral (flexor) surface. Later, the nail fields and their nerve supply will migrate from the tips onto the dorsal surface of each digit.

As the nail fields reach their dorsal position, the epidermis surrounding them forms folds on both sides and proximally. The nail plate and future nail appear, as cells from the proximal nail fold grow over the nail field and become keratinised. Initially, there is a superficial layer of epidermis (eponychium) covering the nail plate, but this degenerates and exposes the plate. Its remnant persists as the cuticle. The fingernails reach the fingertips by Week 32 and the toenails reach the toetips by Week 36. In both cases the nails grow to reach the tips of the digits by birth.

The face of a newborn may be scratched by the nails even before birth.

117. NAILS

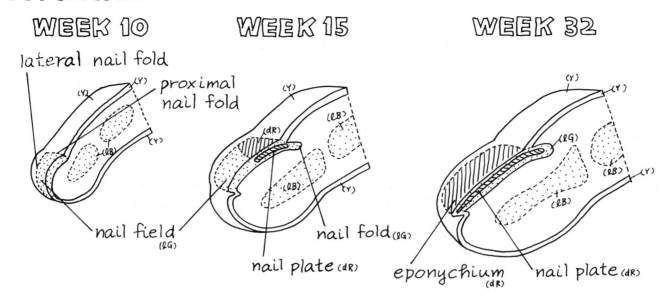

WEEK 10   **WEEK 15**   **WEEK 32**

lateral nail fold

proximal nail fold

nail field (lG)

nail plate (dR)

nail fold (lG)

eponychium (dR)

nail plate (dR)

118. Mammary Glands

In Week 4, a region of thickened ectoderm appears bilaterally in the pectoral region. Then in Week 6, the pectoral thickening enlarges and grows into the underlying mesenchyme. Secondary cords grow out from this area into the surrounding mesenchyme and form lactiferous ducts. During Weeks 32–36, these downgrowths and cords become canalised. The mesenchyme forms the fat and fibrous connective tissue of the gland. At birth, both male and female glands are similar in appearance.

A depressed mammary pit forms in the epidermis above the gland. The nipple forms close to term or in the neonatal period as underlying mesenchyme proliferates below the downgrowths and elevates this area above the adjacent skin.

Anomalies of the Mammary Gland

Supernumerary mammary glands may form anywhere from the pectoral to the inguinal region.

118. MAMMARY GLANDS

STAGE 16 STAGE 19 WEEK 13

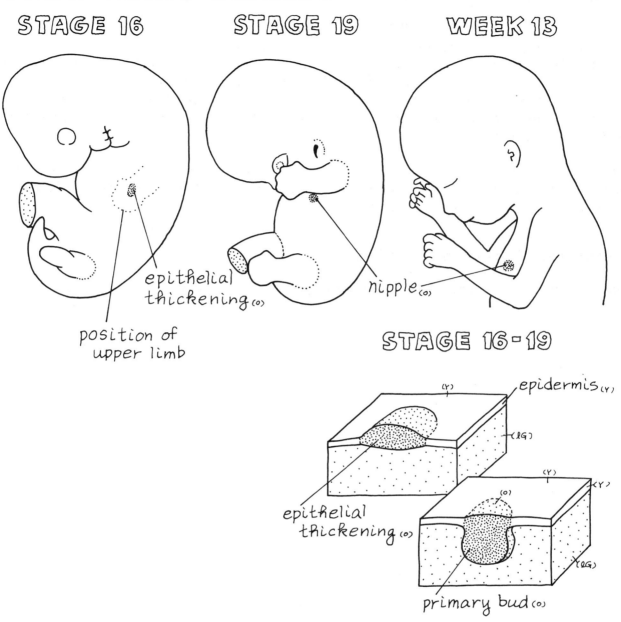

epithelial thickening (o)

nipple (o)

position of upper limb

STAGE 16-19

epidermis (Y)

(Y)

(lG)

epithelial thickening (o)

(o)

(Y)

(lG)

primary bud (o)

WEEK 13 AT TERM

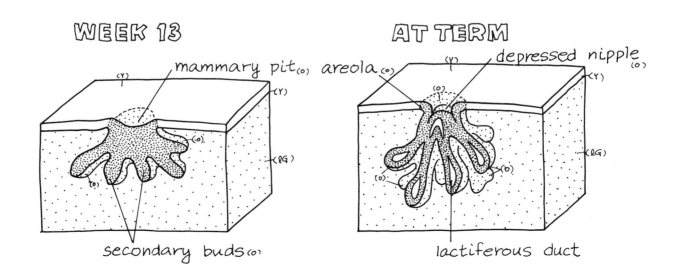

mammary pit (o) areola (o) depressed nipple (o)

(Y) (Y) (Y)

(lG) (lG)

(o) (o)

secondary buds (o) lactiferous duct

119. Teeth

The primordia of both the 20 deciduous teeth and of most of the 32 permanent teeth are present at birth.

All the layers of a tooth are derived from mesenchyme, except for the enamel which is of ectodermal origin. There are three stages of tooth development: the bud stage, the cap stage and the bell stage.

Bud Stage

In Week 6, the oral epithelium thickens to form dental laminae in each jaw. Ten centres appear in each dental lamina for the ten deciduous (milk) teeth in that jaw. In Week 10 the tooth buds of some of the permanent teeth appear lingual to the deciduous tooth buds. The buds of the permanent teeth not present as deciduous teeth develop after birth from prolongations of the dental laminae. The permanent teeth develop similarly to the deciduous teeth.

As not all of the teeth develop at the same time, various stages are present in the mouth. Maturation is most advanced in the midline and then progresses posteriorly in each jaw.

Cap Stage

As the tooth bud grows, it is invaginated by mesenchyme. The bud becomes cap shaped, and because its external portion produces enamel, it is termed the enamel organ. The invaginated mesenchyme is known as the dental papilla and will give rise to the dentin and dental pulp. The cells of the inner enamel epithelium differentiate to form ameloblasts which deposit enamel over the dentin. As the enamel thickens, the ameloblasts migrate towards the outer enamel epithelium.

Bell Stage

At this stage the tooth assumes a bell shape. Two layers differentiate, i.e. the mesenchyme cells in the dental papilla adjacent to the inner enamel epithelium, and the inner enamel epithelium. The mesenchyme adjacent to the inner enamel epithelium differentiates into odontoblasts and deposits pre-dentin which later calcifies and forms dentin. As more dentin accumulates, the odontoblasts migrate towards the centre of the dental papilla leaving cytoplasmic processes (Tomes' processes) embedded in the dentin in their wake.

The cells of the inner enamel epithelium differentiate to form ameloblasts which deposit enamel over the dentin. As the enamel thickens, the ameloblasts migrate towards the outer enamel epithelium.

The root forms when a fold (epithelial root sheath) from the junction of the outer and inner enamel epithelium grows into the adjacent mesenchyme and induces root formation. Odontoblasts adjacent to this sheath produce dentin which reduces the pulp cavity to a narrow root canal containing the vessels and nerves passing to the tooth.

119. TEETH
STAGE 23 (WEEK 8)

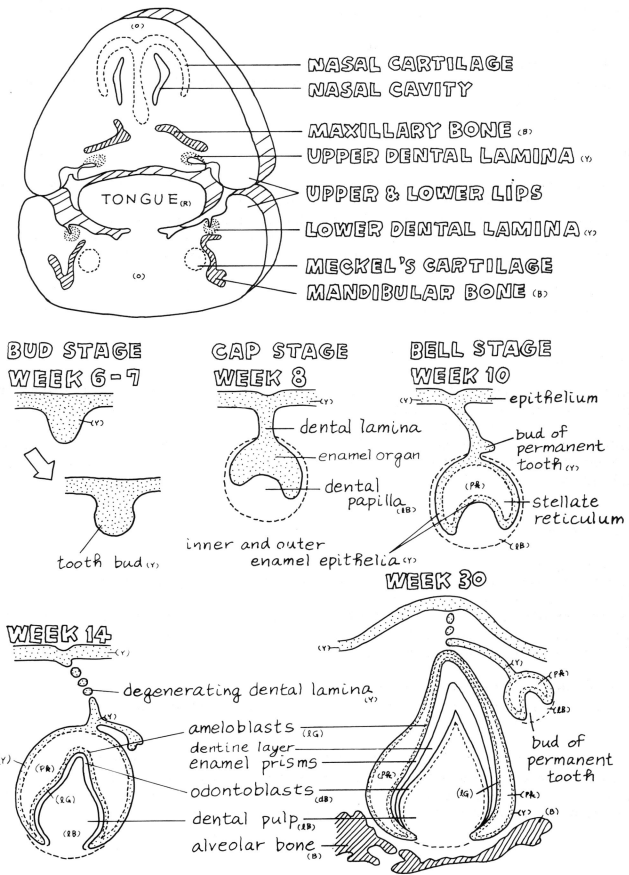

NASAL CARTILAGE

NASAL CAVITY

MAXILLARY BONE (B)

UPPER DENTAL LAMINA (Y)

UPPER & LOWER LIPS

LOWER DENTAL LAMINA (Y)

MECKEL'S CARTILAGE

MANDIBULAR BONE (B)

TONGUE (R)

BUD STAGE WEEK 6-7

tooth bud (Y)

CAP STAGE WEEK 8

dental lamina

enamel organ

dental papilla (lB)

inner and outer enamel epithelia (Y)

BELL STAGE WEEK 10

epithelium

bud of permanent tooth (Y)

stellate reticulum

WEEK 14

degenerating dental lamina (Y)

ameloblasts (lG)

dentine layer

enamel prisms

odontoblasts (dB)

dental pulp (lB)

alveolar bone (B)

WEEK 30

bud of permanent tooth

As the dental sac differentiates, the inner cells form cementoblasts which produce cementum and the outer cells participate in bone formation around the root of the tooth. The dental sac also gives rise to the periodontal ligament which is embedded both in the cementum and the bony alveolus (tooth socket) and holds the tooth in its bony socket.

In the neonate the first teeth to erupt at 6 months are normally the central mandibular incisors.

The length of the developing face in childhood is affected by the development of the teeth and the paranasal sinuses.

Anomalies of Tooth Development

Discoloration of the milk teeth and permanent teeth enamel occurs if tetracyclines are administered to the mother at 18 weeks gestation or later. Excessive fluoride ingested in childhood also causes discoloration.

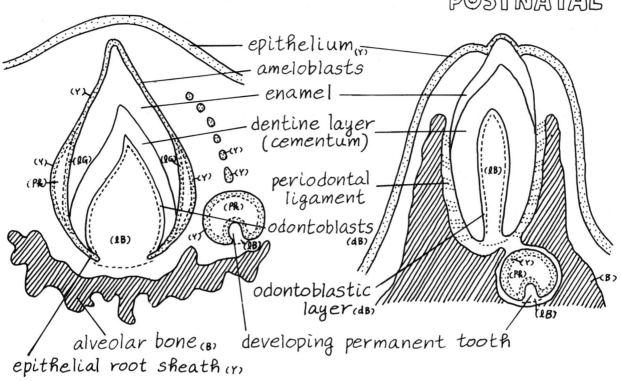

epithelium (Y)
ameloblasts
enamel
dentine layer (cementum)
periodontal ligament
odontoblasts (dB)
odontoblastic layer (dB)
alveolar bone (B)
developing permanent tooth
epithelial root sheath (Y)

5-YEAR OLD

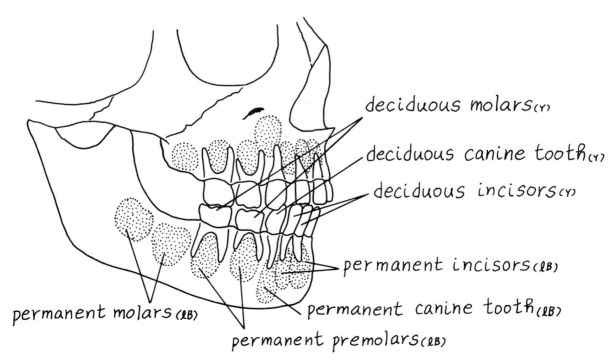

deciduous molars (Y)
deciduous canine tooth (Y)
deciduous incisors (Y)
permanent incisors (lB)
permanent canine tooth (lB)
permanent molars (lB)
permanent premolars (lB)

120. Salivary Glands

The largest pair of salivary glands, the parotids, are ectodermal in origin, while the submandibular and sublingual glands are endodermal in origin. Their different origins are based on their position relative to the oropharyngeal membrane in the future mouth. The parotid and submandibular glands begin to develop before the sublingual glands.

All three pairs develop similarly. The epithelium of the oral cavity forms a solid bud which grows into the underlying mesenchyme. The bud branches to form solid cords with rounded tips. Later these tips will form the acini, while the surrounding mesenchyme forms the capsule and connective tissue of the salivary gland. Later the solid cords develop lumina and ducts.

120. SALIVARY GLANDS
STAGE 14 (WEEK 5)   AT TERM

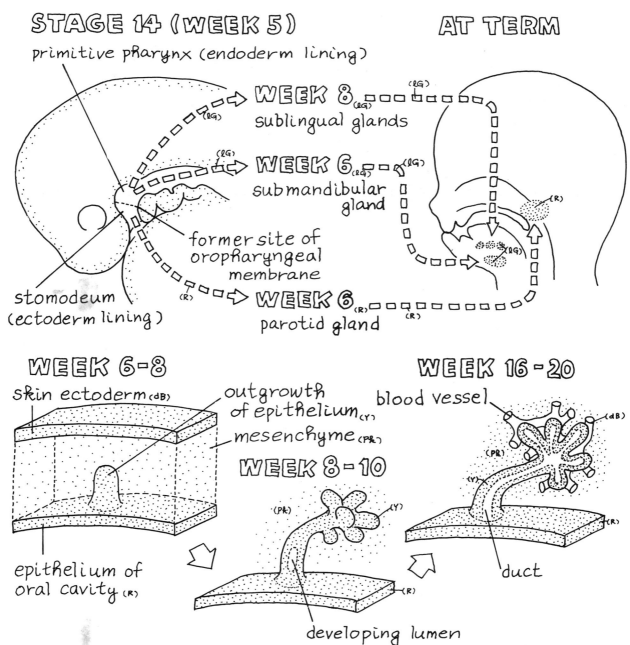

primitive pharynx (endoderm lining)

WEEK 8 (ℓG)
sublingual glands

WEEK 6 (ℓG)
submandibular gland

former site of oropharyngeal membrane

stomodeum (ectoderm lining)

WEEK 6 (R)
parotid gland

WEEK 6-8

skin ectoderm (dB)

outgrowth of epithelium (Y)

mesenchyme (Pk)

WEEK 8-10

epithelium of oral cavity (R)

developing lumen

WEEK 16-20

blood vessel

duct

121. Congenital Malformations

A congenital malformation or anomaly is a microscopic or macroscopic defect resulting from defective development. These anomalies are the results of genetic factors, environmental agents, and multifactorial causes. Approximately 3% of neonates have major congenital malformations. A defect may be minor or major, single or in multiples. Most major defects occur in early embryonic development and these embryos usually abort naturally.

Periods of Sensitivity

In the course of development, there are periods of sensitivity for each tissue, organ, or system. During these times, the tissue is at its most vulnerable to the actions of teratogens, which are agents that bring about congenital defects. In the first 2 weeks of development, teratogens usually cause embryonic death. During the embryonic period (15–60 days) they may cause major congenital defects, and during the fetal period they may result in structural and functional anomalies.

121. CONGENITAL MALFORMATIONS: PERIODS OF SENSITIVITY

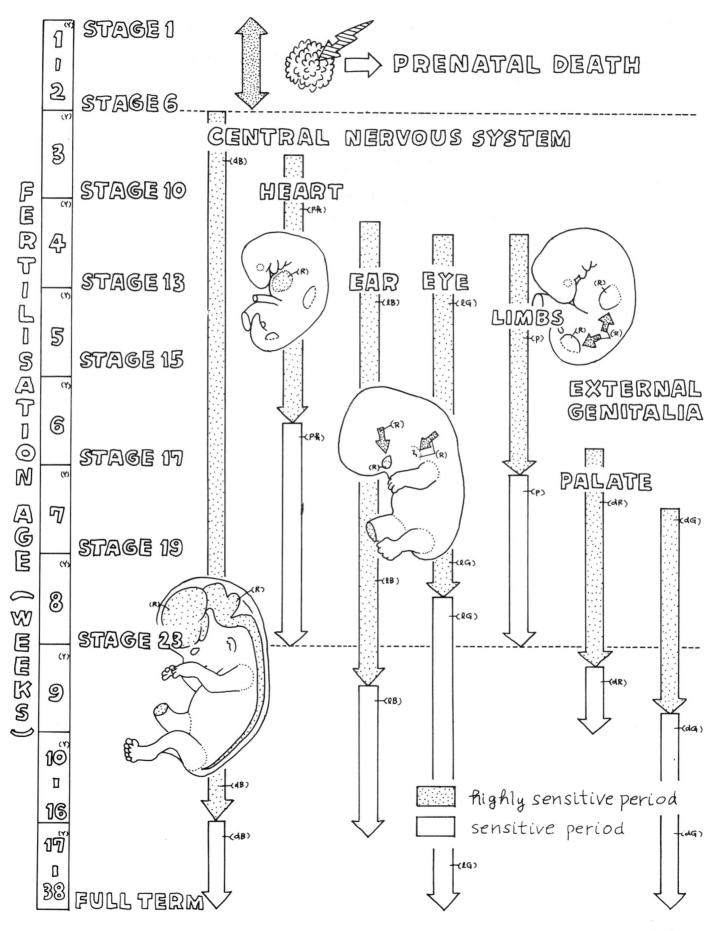

PRENATAL DEATH

CENTRAL NERVOUS SYSTEM

HEART

EAR   EYE

LIMBS

EXTERNAL GENITALIA

PALATE

- highly sensitive period
- sensitive period

303

Genetic Factors

Genetic factors are the most important known cause of congenital malformations. Chromosomes may be altered structurally when affected by environmental factors. If a chromosome breaks, there may be several outcomes: a piece of chromosome may be lost (deletion); a piece of chromosome may be transferred to a non-homologous chromosome (translocation); a piece of chromosome may become reversed (inversion); or a portion of a chromosome may be duplicated (duplication). If the centromere divides transversely instead of longitudinally (isochromosome), this can also result in abnormalities.

Abnormal numbers of chromosomes (aneuploidy) may also be associated with congenital abnormalities. The condition can result from defective chromosome or chromatid separation (non-disjunction) during the first or second meiotic division in gametogenesis. Loss of one member of a chromosome pair (monosomy) appears to be lethal in humans if it affects an autosome. Gain of a chromosome gives trisomy. Down's syndrome is referred to as trisomy 21, which denotes three number 21 chromosomes. Trisomy 13 and 18 are less common. The occurrence of autosomal trisomies increases with maternal age. There are many known abnormalities of the sex chromosome. Turner's syndrome is characterised by the presence of only one sex chromosome (XO). Trisomy of sex chromosomes can result in XXY (Klinefelter's syndrome), XYY, or XXX individuals. Combinations involving four or five X chromosomes have been reported.

Mutant Genes

Malformations can be caused by mutant genes. These are genes which have undergone a change or a loss in function. Often this is a result of environmental factors such as ionising radiation or carcinogenic (cancer inducing) agents. To be inherited, mutations must be present in the germ line.

Environmental Agents

Environmental teratogens include drugs, chemicals, infectious agents, radiation and mechanical factors. Examples of drugs include alcohol, thalidomide, tetracyclines and most anticoagulants. Chemicals which disturb normal embryogenesis include excess retinoic acid (vitamin A), iodides, and mercury. Drugs and chemicals together are responsible for less than 2% of recorded congenital malformations. Infectious agents known to cross the placenta include the rubella virus (German measles), varicella zoster virus (chickenpox) and cytomegalovirus. Ionising radiation in large doses has been shown to produce congenital malformations. Mechanical factors can contribute to postural defects. For example, a significant lack of amniotic fluid (oligohydramnios) can lead to foot deformities.

Multifactorial Causes

Most congenital malformations are due to a combination of a genetic predisposition and environmental factors.

Unknown Causes

More than half of congenital malformations have no known cause.

▷ GENETIC FACTORS : 15 %

○ CHROMOSOMAL ABNORMALITIES

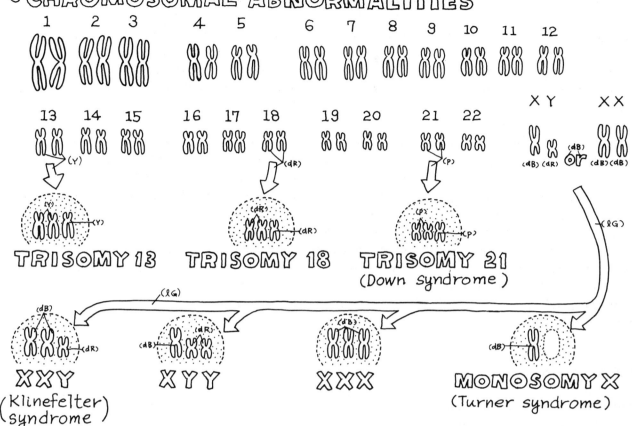

TRISOMY 13   TRISOMY 18   TRISOMY 21
(Down syndrome)

XXY   XYY   XXX   MONOSOMY X
(Klinefelter   (Turner syndrome)
syndrome)

○ MUTANT GENES
⇨ INHERITED MALFORMATION

▷ ENVIRONMENTAL AGENTS : 10 %

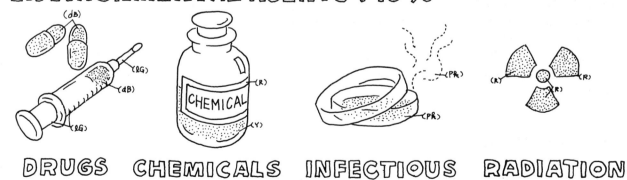

DRUGS   CHEMICALS   INFECTIOUS   RADIATION
AGENTS   etc.

▷ MULTIFACTORIAL CAUSES : 25 %
▷ UNKNOWN CAUSES : > 50 %

References

AREY, L. B. (1974), *Developmental Anatomy: A Textbook and Laboratory Manual of Embryology*, Revised 7th Edition; W.B. Saunders Co., Philadelphia pp 1–612.

AUSTIN, C.R. (1989), *Human Embryos*; Oxford University Press, Oxford, pp 1–163.

BLECHSCHMIDT, E. (1977), *The Beginnings of Human Life*; Heidelberg Science Library, Springer-Verlag, Berlin pp 1–128.

DAVIES, J. (1963), *Human Developmental Anatomy*; The Ronald Press, New York, pp 1–298.

ENGLAND, M.A. (1983), *A Colour Atlas of Life Before Birth: Normal Fetal Development*; Wolfe Medical Publications Ltd, London, pp 1–216.

ENGLAND, M.A. (1989), *Picture Tests in Embryology*; Wolfe Medical Publications Ltd, London, pp 1–128.

FITZGERALD, M.J.T. (1978), *Human Embryology: A Regional Approach;* Harper and Row, Hagerstown, Maryland, pp 1–205.

GASSER, R.F. (1975), *Atlas of Human Embryos*; Harper and Row, London, pp 1–318.

HAINES, R.W. and MOHIUDDIN, A. (1972), *Handbook of Human Embryology,* 5th Edition; Churchill Livingstone, London, pp 1–252.

HAMILTON, W.J. and MOSSMAN, H.W. (1972), *Human Embryology: Prenatal Development of Form and Function*, 4th Edition; W. Heffer and Sons Ltd, Cambridge, pp 1–646.

GILBERT, S.G. (1989), *Pictorial Human Embryology*; University of Washington Press, London, pp 3–172.

JOHNSON, D.R. (1986), *The Genetics of the Skeleton, Animal Models of Skeletal Development*; Clarendon Press, Oxford, pp 1–407.

JOHNSON, K.E. (1988), *Human Developmental Anatomy*; John Wiley & Sons Inc., New York, pp 1–447.

MARIN-PADILLA, M. (1983), Structural Organization of the Human Cerebral Cortex Prior to the Appearance of the Cortical Plate. *Anatomy & Embryology*, **168:** 21–40.

MARIN-PADILLA, M. (1988), Early Ontogenesis of the Human Cerebral Cortex. In: Jones, E.G., Peters, A. (eds)*Cerebral Cortex: Cellular Components of the Cerebral Cortex* **VII**: pp 1–17, Plenum Press, New York.

MOORE, K.L. (1988), *The Developing Human: Clinically Orientated Embryology*, 4th Edition; W.B. Saunders Co., pp 1–462.

NISHIMURA, H. (Ed) (1983), *Atlas of Human Prenatal Histology*; Igaku-Shoin, Tokyo, pp 1–316.

O'RAHILLY, R. and MULLER, F. (1987), *Developmental Stages in Human Embryos*; Carnegie Institution of Washington Publication **637**: 1–306.

PANSKY B. (1982), *Review of Medical Embryology*; MacMillan, New York, pp 1–527.

PATTEN, B.M. (1946), *Human Embryology;* The Blakiston Company Inc., New York, pp 1–776.

SADLER, T.W. (1990), *Langman's Medical Embryology*, 6th Edition; Williams & Wilkins, London, pp 1–411.

WILLIAMS, P.L., WARWICK, R., DYSON, M. and BANNISTER, L.H. (Eds) (1989), *Gray's Anatomy*, 37th Edition; Churchill Livingstone, Edinburgh, pp 1–1598.

WILLIAMS, P.L. and WENDELL-SMITH, C.P. (1969), *Basic Human Embryology*; Pitman Medical, Edinburgh, pp 1–162.

Index